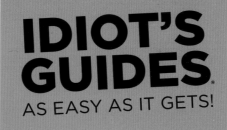

IDIOT'S GUIDES.
AS EASY AS IT GETS!

Stretching

by Melanie Roberts, MS, and Stephanie Kaiser, MS

ALPHA

A member of Penguin Group (USA) Inc.

ALPHA BOOKS

Published by Penguin Group (USA) Inc.

Penguin Group (USA) Inc., 375 Hudson Street, New York, New York 10014, USA · Penguin Group (Canada), 90 Eglinton Avenue East, Suite 700, Toronto, Ontario M4P 2Y3, Canada (a division of Pearson Penguin Canada Inc.) · Penguin Books Ltd., 80 Strand, London WC2R 0RL, England · Penguin Ireland, 25 St. Stephen's Green, Dublin 2, Ireland (a division of Penguin Books Ltd.) · Penguin Group (Australia), 250 Camberwell Road, Camberwell, Victoria 3124, Australia (a division of Pearson Australia Group Pty. Ltd.) · Penguin Books India Pvt. Ltd., 11 Community Centre, Panchsheel Park, New Delhi—110 017, India · Penguin Group (NZ), 67 Apollo Drive, Rosedale, North Shore, Auckland 1311, New Zealand (a division of Pearson New Zealand Ltd.) · Penguin Books (South Africa) (Pty.) Ltd., 24 Sturdee Avenue, Rosebank, Johannesburg 2196, South Africa · Penguin Books Ltd., Registered Offices: 80 Strand, London WC2R 0RL, England

Copyright © 2013 by Penguin Group (USA) Inc.

International Standard Book Number: 978-1-61564-421-6
Library of Congress Catalog Card Number: 2013940219

15   14   13   8   7   6   5   4   3   2   1

Interpretation of the printing code: The rightmost number of the first series of numbers is the year of the book's printing; the rightmost number of the second series of numbers is the number of the book's printing. For example, a printing code of 13-1 shows that the first printing occurred in 2013.

Publisher: *Mike Sanders*
Executive Managing Editor: *Billy Fields*
Acquisitions Editor: *Brook Farling*
Development Editor: *John Etchison*

Senior Production Editor: *Janette Lynn*
Cover Designer: *William Thomas*
Book Designer: *Kurt Owens, Rebecca Batchelor*
Photographer: *Mark Lee*

Contents

Core 97

Hips 107

3 Stretching Routines 168

Introduction

Congratulations on taking the first step toward improving your flexibility and well-being by opening this book! Whether you're new to stretching or have years of experience, this book will provide you the tools and motivation you need to achieve your fitness goals. Use this book as your trusted guide for designing your very own flexibility program based on your needs and your schedule.

Stretching is easy, it's relaxing, and it pays big dividends. Most of you don't need this book to tell you that your flexibility changes over time. And we don't mean for the better. Without giving it much thought, our movements throughout each day remain fairly consistent. Our muscles and joints become comfortable within a defined range of motion, and when something out of the ordinary is required, muscle strains and injuries won't be far behind.

Flexibility is what allows you to move freely, balance yourself in changing situations, and take on new challenges as they are presented. The added bonus from flexibility training is that you feel the results and see your improvements quickly. You just need to get started!

How to Use This Book

Part 1 covers all the basics of stretching and then some. More than just how to put together a safe and effective stretching routine, you'll learn how to maximize your flexibility by adding dynamic movements and foam roller techniques. You'll know what areas to target after scoring yourself on seven critical flexibility tests. There are many more tips and tools to help you make the most of your time and keep you in top shape.

In Part 2, we show you how to complete a variety of stretches. Photos and detailed descriptions will walk you through stretches for every part of the body. Each exercise has a full explanation with photos and numbered steps to guide you correctly through the stretch for the best results possible. Foam rolling and dynamic stretches are presented first, followed by static stretches. Also included are modifications that can be used to alter the intensity and create a more or less challenging movement when needed. Other items to look out for in this part are caution sidebars to help you avoid potential injury, and tip sidebars to help you get the maximum benefit from the stretches.

Part 3, the final part, contains a variety of routines geared toward sports and daily activities and can be adapted to a variety of needs. Look to these routines for ideas to supplement your own personalized exercise program. All the stretches are detailed in Part 2, so you can reference these when trying a routine.

Acknowledgments

While not every person who is responsible for the knowledge presented in this book can be listed in the space provided, we would like to thank several people who made the work a reality. We thank the staff of the National Institute for Fitness and Sport for their endless knowledge, passion, and support. It's an honor to represent all of you. A special thanks to our modest-in-real-life models Crystal Belen, Michael Hoess, Josh Jones, Alan Mikesky, Tasha Nichols, and Susan Huppert, for showing what great flexibility looks like. A thank you to photographer Mark Lee, for capturing all the great images you will see in this book. And our sincerest thanks to acquisitions editor Brook Farling, development editor John Etchison, and the entire team at Alpha Books for shaping and creating this book.

Part 1

Flexibility Fundamentals

Part 1 provides you with the practical knowledge and useful resources you'll need for greater flexibility and easier movement. We cover all the basic elements of stretching, such as the best time to stretch, how long to hold a stretch, and how far and how frequently you should stretch.

Then we take you a step further with easy-to-follow techniques that will take your stretching program to a higher level. You'll learn about dynamic movements and Active Isolated Stretching, and why your muscles respond differently to these techniques compared to static stretching.

There's also a flexibility test and scorecard that provides an excellent starting point so you can assess your mobility strengths and weaknesses and measure your progress over time. In addition, you'll learn how a few simple tools and props can greatly improve the way you stretch and the benefits you receive.

So don't wait—get started now on your path to greater flexibility and easier movement.

How to Get the Most from This Book

This book provides a wide variety of stretches, but not all of them are appropriate for everyone. To ensure that a program is safe and effective for you, talk to your doctor, physical therapist, or an exercise professional about which exercises are best suited to help you reach your fitness goals. This is especially true if you've had an injury or surgery to a joint, or any neck or back problems.

There are several common themes throughout this book. Some you might be familiar with and others may be new to you. With so many stretches to choose from, it's important to know how to tailor a program that's right for you. After all, you'll be the one to pick and choose the stretches from this book to build a safe and effective program. It's not complicated, but it is important to know the following basics.

Warm-up: Start every flexibility session with a warm-up to increase your core body temperature. When you break a sweat, you know you're there! Brisk walking, light jogging, rowing, and biking are all good examples. A good warm-up may take 5 to 10 minutes.

Dynamic movements: After a good warm-up, complete the dynamic movements for each joint and the muscles that will be used in the activity you're about to begin. Your goal is to mimic the movements and prepare the specific muscles you're going to engage in your activity. Always complete dynamic movements before static stretching and before your activity if you're preparing your muscles for a workout or an athletic performance. Dynamic movements are the perfect way to improve your flexibility, balance, coordination, and strength. These movements give you the best "bang for your buck" and maximize your time.

> **CAUTION:** Never try to stretch a cold muscle! Start every exercise or flexibility session with a gentle warm-up. Gradually boosting your heart rate over 5 to 10 minutes increases blood flow and muscle temperature. This allows your muscles to move more like a soft rubber band. Not only are you reducing your chance of a muscle strain, but your muscles might recover faster with less chance of soreness.

Static stretches: These are best done after a workout—or if flexibility training *is* the workout, the static stretches are completed after the warm-up and dynamic movements. Don't expect to perform every stretch as depicted, but focus on posture, breathing, and correct form. Stay in a pain-free range of motion and your joints will respond by increasing their mobility over time. It's important to not ignore the stretches you find most challenging, as those are the very stretches that may be limiting your mobility the most. Mark the most challenging stretches, and be sure they get your best effort and extra time until they're no longer the weak link in your chain of movement.

The dynamic and active warm-up movements outlined in Parts 2 and 3 are key to your long-term flexibility gains. They not only open your joints and stretch your muscles, they activate your central nervous system so your muscles can receive the message your brain is sending. Continue to grow your list of dynamic movements that mimic your sport or activities.

Foam rolling: Once you try this, you may want to do it all the time! Rolling, a.k.a. "my cheap massage," is a great way to help your muscles recover, as well as release their tension and gain elasticity. Using the foam roller can be uncomfortable when you first try it, just like a deep massage. Be patient. After several sessions with the foam roller, your muscles will respond and you will almost feel them loosen up. You can try rolling your muscles before a workout, after a workout, or even while watching television.

Stretching Tips to Remember

Don't use stretching as a warm-up. Stretching a cold muscle is like flipping a frozen rubber band.

Don't aim for pain. If you lengthen the muscle too far, too fast, or hold for too long, your muscle will contract to try to protect itself and defeat your stretching efforts. See the following "Be Aware of the Stretch Reflex" section.

Stick with it. The good news about stretching is that changes in flexibility happen relatively quickly. The bad news is they leave just as fast. Once you feel you've achieved good flexibility, you should be able to maintain it with three or four sessions per week, depending on your other activities.

Focus on your tight areas. While it might be tempting to do only the "easy" stretches that feel good, your greatest gains will come from stretching the areas you find most challenging.

Incorporate movement. Go beyond the dynamic stretches and yoga poses in this book, and try a yoga or tai chi class. If you're preparing for a specific sport, you'll want to expand your library of dynamic movements to mimic the moves required for the activity. Using all your muscles together, the same way you move in life and sport, is the most effective training of all.

Don't bounce. Not to be confused with dynamic movement, bouncing can lead to tissue damage and the counterproductive stretch reflex. Keep the stretches controlled and smooth.

Be Aware of the Stretch Reflex

The stretch reflex is a protective mechanism within the muscles that helps to prevent overstretching and muscle or tendon injury. If when performing a stretch you try to lengthen the muscle too far or too fast, or hold a stretch too long, your muscle will contract to protect itself. Since a muscle cannot stretch and contract at the same time, activating the stretch reflex will prevent gains in flexibility. As a general rule, if a stretch brings a grimace to your face, you've probably activated the stretch reflex. This might feel as if you've hit an endpoint in the stretch rather than a cushioned landing.

Stay Flexible, Move Easier

Your body is designed to move. It thrives on reaching, pushing, pulling, bending, climbing, and jumping. Your body grows stronger and your senses awaken when your muscles are pumping, blood rushes through your body, oxygen fills your lungs, and your mind is engaged. So whether you enjoy dancing, running, walking, gardening, athletics, or yoga, it's important you do something that nourishes your body with the power of movement. This book is meant to help everyone get started with gentle stretches that can be stepping-stones to a more active lifestyle.

Flexibility is not a goal to be achieved and then forgotten. To maintain flexibility, you must continue to teach your body movements that push you to new heights. The information about what is best for your body can be overwhelming and difficult to decipher, but you can rise above the uncertainty by staying focused on three basic principles:

1. You are in charge of taking care of your body.

2. Your body needs good fuel, regular exercise, preventive maintenance, and lots of TLC.

3. If you listen to your body, it will tell you how well you're doing so you can adjust your plan accordingly.

While there's no doubt that flexibility is essential to mobility, balance, athletic performance, and injury prevention, it's important to know what flexibility is. Flexibility is the ability to move a joint through its full range of motion (ROM). Flexibility training shouldn't be confused with simply stretching, though. Many times stretching is no more than a kind of "spot check" to see how well you're moving, like lifting your heel to your buttocks just before going on a quick run.

Flexibility training, on the other hand, is the thoughtful art of putting together dynamic movements, static stretches, and other techniques you'll learn here as a way to achieve maximum function and ROM in your joints. Done properly, flexibility training will actually increase the elasticity of your muscles and the tendons that connect muscles to bones. Think of flexibility as the desired outcome and stretching as the means to achieve it.

The Different Types of Stretching

There are a variety of stretching categories to choose from, and each serves its own purpose in helping you achieve your goals. Any apprehension you might have about learning a new way of stretching will quickly disappear as you notice almost immediate gains in your flexibility. Each of these techniques has something to offer everyone, from beginner to veteran. Each technique complements the others and has its place in your regimen. What varies is the intensity and duration for each stretch. Whatever your starting point, you can count on gains from all types of stretching.

Dynamic Stretching

Dynamic stretching involves active movements that are generally done prior to an activity or moving into other forms of stretching. The unique advantage of dynamic stretching is that it moves your joints and recruits your muscles the same way you use them in real life. Whether you're stepping out of the car or running around the track, your muscles move in incredibly complex patterns. Aim to increase your menu of dynamic stretches over time to counter your tightest areas and the muscles most important to your activities. When developing a warm-up program and considering the active stretches to include, be sure to choose dynamic stretches for each major muscle group you'll be using during your activity. Complete 8 to 12 repetitions of the movement before moving to the next.

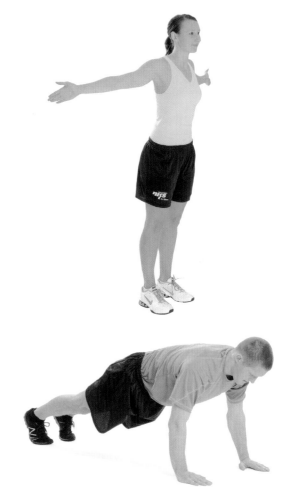

Static Stretching

The bulk of this book describes static stretches. These are the stretches you're most likely familiar with, and the stretches you hold as explained later. Your body isn't in motion when you complete a static stretch. It's best to static stretch at the end of an activity or after you've completed your dynamic stretches, so as not to stretch cold muscles. You'll receive the greatest benefits from these stretches with the muscles already warmed up.

Be sure to focus on areas where you feel the most tightness, and experiment with as many different stretches as you feel comfortable with. You'll want to be familiar with as many stretches as possible so you have various options based on your changing needs. When planning your stretches around an activity, think of the major muscle groups you'll be using and be sure to pick a few stretches that target those areas.

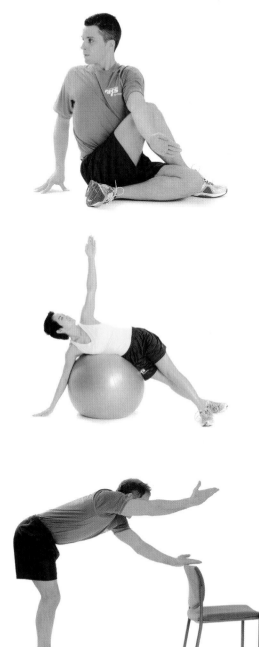

Contract and Relax/AIS Stretching

Active Isolated Stretching (AIS) is a technique that incorporates a gentle external pressure, applied with your hand or a rope, intended to reprogram your nervous system with a new range of motion. It's also known as contract and relax stretching. It works by pairing up opposite muscles and allowing one muscle to relax its opposite contracts.

Generally, this type of stretch is assisted by a rope, as seen in this book, or by another individual. Use the assistance to increase your normal range of motion for 1 or 2 seconds (don't hold for longer or the stretch reflex will be activated), then relax for 5 to 10 seconds, and repeat the sequence 8 to 10 times for 1 or 2 sets. Exhale during the stretch phase and inhale on the return phase. Consider using this type of stretching on all the major muscle groups to see immense gains in your range of motion.

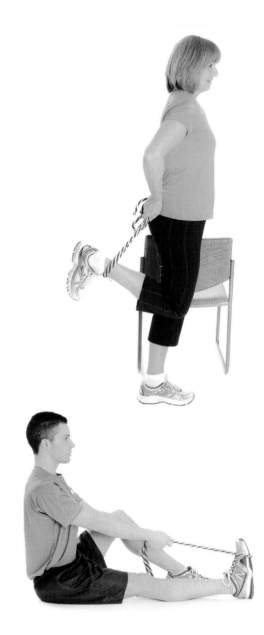

Building Your Stretching Program

The first step in choosing the correct stretches to include in your program is to identify your goal. Knowing what you wish to gain from the routine will help lead you in the right direction when creating your plan. In Part 3, we've created routines geared toward common activities. These routines focus on the muscles that are used most or are commonly injured during the particular activity. Look to these for an excellent example of how to structure your own routine, or simply pick the one that best suits your goals.

Whether your goal is to get through daily activities, improve athletic performance, or release muscle tension, it's important to consider the nuts and bolts that contribute to a successful program. Although your own reason for starting a flexibility program may be different from someone else's, the programs are built on the same fundamental elements needed to improve flexibility. The reality is that there's a right way and a wrong way to build a stretching program. This section will teach you the keys to building one the right way!

One of the nice things about stretching is that you can stretch almost anywhere and anytime! It's important to keep this in mind, especially for those who are on the go and find it difficult to find the spare time. Ideally, it would be nice to have a solid 15 to 30 minute block of time to dedicate to your routine most days of the week. This isn't always feasible with a busy schedule, but exercising for even a few minutes can provide big benefits.

If you sit at a desk for much of the day, consider choosing stretches that can be done while seated or within the area of your work space. On the contrary, if you spend most of your day standing, choose stretches that can be done while you're standing and consider the space and objects around you that can be implemented in your routine. Pausing for a few minutes here and there, waiting in a long line at the grocery store, or finding a 5 or 10 minute break at work are examples of excellent opportunities to squeeze in a few minutes of stretching!

Stretching the Right Way

To get the full benefit from your effort to improve your flexibility, you should hold static stretches for 10 to 30 seconds. First, it's important to understand the difference between feeling tension and feeling pain. Applying slight tension to feel the stretch is a good thing, but feeling pain is bad. A stretch should *never* feel painful! Stay inside your comfort zone! If a stretch is causing pain, you should back off and see if completing the stretch to a lesser degree is doable. If there's still pain, you should avoid it and consider checking with your doctor or therapist in case there's an injury.

On the other hand, once you reach the place during a static stretch where you feel gentle tension in the muscle, you should hold the stretch. At this point, you're in a position where increased flexibility and range of motion can be attained.

The amount of time to hold a stretch and how many times you repeat the stretch will vary based on time and conditioning level. The following are good general principles to achieve the best results:

- Beginners should start out on the lower end, holding a stretch for 10 to 20 seconds and repeating the stretch 1 to 3 times.
- Those who are at a more intermediate level can hold for 20 to 30 seconds and repeat the stretch 2 to 4 times.
- Advanced exercisers can hold the stretch for 30 to 40 seconds, repeating 3 to 5 times and adjusting the tension of the stretch as you move through the ROM.

Another important piece to consider is breathing technique. First and foremost, never hold your breath while you're stretching. For some, the natural instinct is to hold the stretch and forget to breathe, tensing up the muscles and often cutting the stretch short.

For the most part, think about keeping your breathing pattern the same. When completing longer holds, an option is to take deep breaths and move deeper into the stretch. For example, if you're doing a seated hamstring stretch, you might take a few deep breaths during the stretch and reach a little farther toward your toes each time you exhale. Breathing also plays a key role in relaxation stretches. Using the breath as a rhythm helps you relax into the stretch.

Stretching the Wrong Way

While we've already discussed that feeling pain in the muscle and not breathing during stretching are counterproductive, there are other things that should also be avoided. One of the most important rules is to never static stretch a cold muscle. This being said, you should always do an active warm-up before you begin static stretching. This could be a short walk or jog or a routine of dynamic stretches prior to a workout; or you could wait to complete your stretching routine after a workout. Each section in Part 2 starts with a foam roller and/or dynamic stretch that can also be performed before starting static stretches.

Another rule to remember is you should never "bounce" as you're holding a stretch. This can lead to injury to the muscles or connective tissues. Dynamic stretching can provide superior results and is considered much safer. Don't look at stretching as a way to heal an injury. If you feel like you've injured a muscle, consult with a doctor before beginning a stretching routine. Overstretching too soon after some injuries can extend your recovery time.

The Importance of Good Posture

Good posture is one of the most important and overlooked elements of successful stretching. It not only serves an aesthetic purpose, but good posture aids breathing and physical health, and prevents joint and soft tissue damage.

It's important to keep a neutral spine while stretching. It's often easy to arch your back or strain your neck to complete a stretch, but the reality is that you're compromising the stretch and placing a strain on your joints.

The following figure shows what good standing posture looks like. Notice that the hips, shoulders, and spine are all aligned and vertical. This is often referred to as "standing tall." Next, some key appearances of poor posture are pictured and described next. Maintaining good posture during the stretches will be reinforced many times throughout this book as a reminder of its importance.

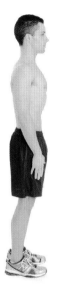

Good Posture

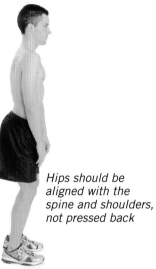

Anterior Pelvic Tilt

Hips should be aligned with the spine and shoulders, not pressed back

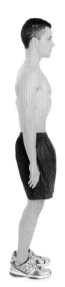

Posterior Pelvic Tilt

Hips should be aligned with the spine and shoulders, not pulled forward

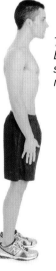
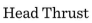

Head Thrust

The neck should be aligned with the spine and shoulders, not pressed forward

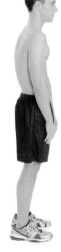

Rounded Shoulders

Shoulders should be pulled back, not rounded forward

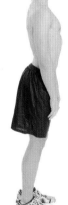

Lordosis

The low back should not be curved inward, but rather aligned with the rest of the spine

Testing Your Flexibility

Testing your flexibility is an important first step in planning your stretching program. These simple tests not only show you what areas are too tight to allow normal range of motion, they can also indicate when a muscle is too loose and allows too much range of motion. Too short and you will not have movement without compensation; too long and you will not have the necessary strength and stability in the joint.

Every person has unique flexibility needs and potential. There's no definitive marker for how much flexibility you should have for every test. Rather, use the following tests as a gauge to locate problem areas and to measure your progress over time. Record your test scores in your initial evaluation and again at regular intervals, such as every 4 or 8 weeks.

Each test begins with a simple description, followed by starting position, the movement, and then recommended stretches you can find in Part 2.

Complete as many of the tests as possible, as flexibility is specific to each joint, and determining your flexibility in a few joints is not an indicator of flexibility in others.

> **CAUTION:** These flexibility tests are intended to be used only as a guide. If you experience pain or have restricted movements or extreme hypermobility, seek the care of a medical doctor, physical therapist, or exercise specialist.

Trunk Rotation

Starting position: Draw a straight vertical line on a wall. Stand with your back to the wall and centered in front of the line. Position yourself arm's length away with your feet shoulder width apart.

Movement: Extend your right arm directly in front and parallel to the floor. Rotate your trunk to your right and try to touch the wall behind you with your fingertips. You can rotate your shoulders, hips, and knees as long as your feet don't move. Repeat with the left side.

Stretches: Half Kneeling Dowel Twist; Kneeling Rotation; Spinal Rotation

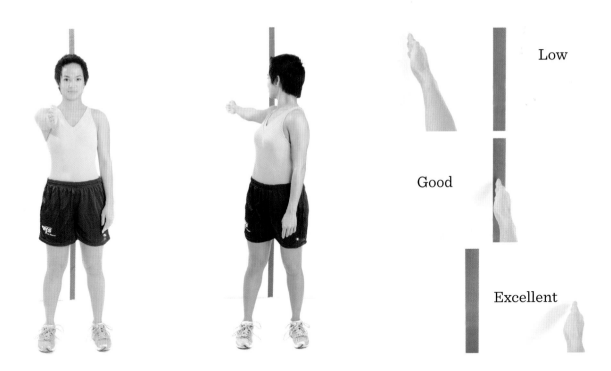

Low

Good

Excellent

Parallel Squat

Starting Position: Stand with feet shoulder width apart and weight evenly distributed through the entire foot.

Movement: Slowly squat as low as possible, but not below parallel. Lower your hips as if you're sitting in a chair. Keep your head neutral and eyes focused forward. Stop if your shoulders go beyond your knees, your knees travel beyond your toes, or your thighs reach parallel. ***Note:*** *This is one of the more difficult movements, as it involves multiple joints. Make a note on your scorecard if you needed to make a modification in order to execute the movement properly.*

Stretches: Forward Lunge; Over and Under Medicine Ball Squat; Standing Calf Stretch

MODIFICATION: If you can't complete this test without bending at the waist, modify by lifting your heels ½ inch to 1 inch by standing on a board, widening your stance, or extending your arms horizontally in front.

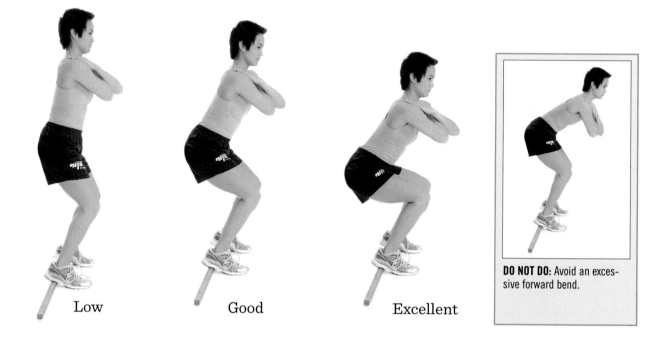

Low   Good   Excellent

DO NOT DO: Avoid an excessive forward bend.

Shoulder Mobility

Starting Position: Stand with your feet shoulder width apart and maintain good posture throughout the movement.

Movement: Raise your left arm, bend your elbow, and reach down across your back as far as possible. At the same time, extend your right down and behind your back, trying to bring your elbow across your back. Try to cross your fingers, upper hand over lower hand. Repeat with your arms in the opposite position.

Stretches: Behind Back Shoulder Reach; Overhead Triceps Rope Stretch; Arm Circles; Kneeling Reach, Roll, and Lift

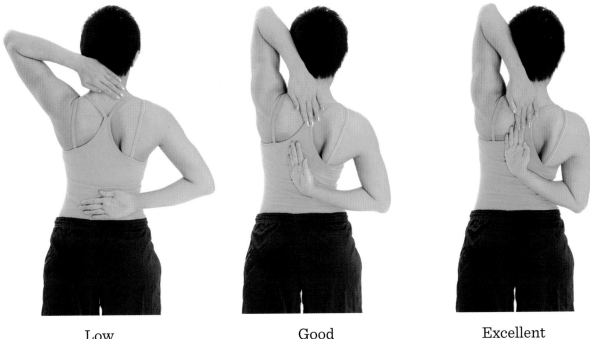

Low   Good   Excellent

Back Extension

Starting Position: Lie on your front with your arms to your side and palms up.

Movement: Slowly raise your torso as high as possible. Keep your head neutral and eyes focused forward.

Stretches: Lying Chest Lift (Cobra); Back Extension on Stability Ball; Cat and Camel

Start

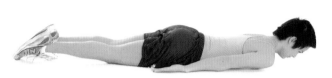

Low

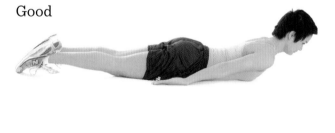

Good

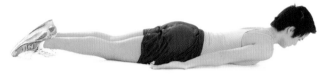

Excellent

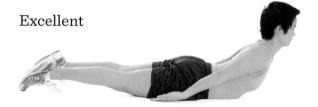

Hip Rotation

Starting Position: Lie on your back with your hips and knees bent at 90 degrees. Arms are fully extended with palms up.

Movement: With your legs together, lower your legs to the floor to the left. Return to center and repeat to the right. Stop the rotation if either shoulder lifts or loses contact with the floor.

Stretches: Standing One Leg Rotation; Iron Cross; Lying Single Leg Crossover

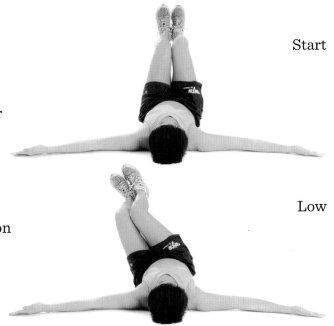

Start

Low

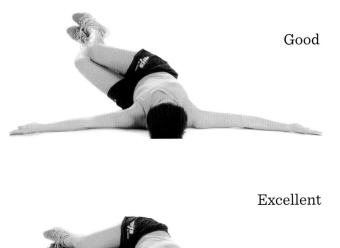

Good

Excellent

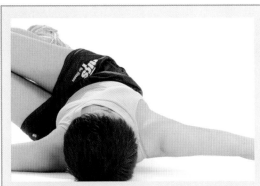

DO NOT DO: Don't lift your should off of the ground when performing this test.

Straight Leg Raise

Starting Position: Lie on your back with arms at your sides and palms facing up.

Movement: Raise one leg with the knee completely straight and ankle at 90 degrees. Repeat with the opposite leg. Be sure to keep your abdominal muscles contracted and the small of your back pressed into the floor throughout the movement.

Stretches: Hamstring Front Leg Swing; Hamstring Rope Stretch; Standing One Leg Hamstring Stretch; Single Knee to Chest

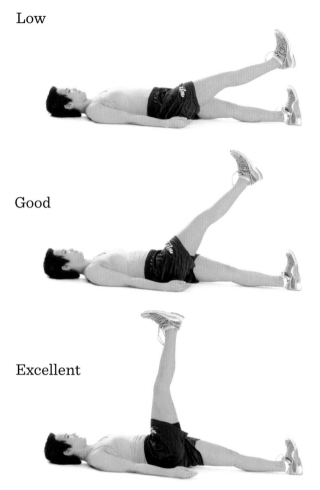

Low

Good

Excellent

Sit and Reach

Starting Position: Sit up tall on the floor with your legs straight and knees flat against the floor. Toes are pointed upward. Extend your arms with one hand on top of the other.

Movement: Slowly reach forward as far as possible while keeping your back flat and head in a neutral position. Exhale as you bend forward. Don't bounce or thrust forward to reach further.

Stretches: Seated Hamstring Stretch; Double Knees to Chest; IT Band and Glute Rope Stretch

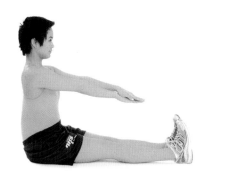

Start

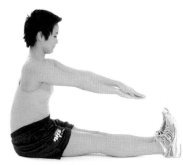

Low

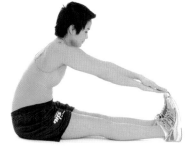

Good

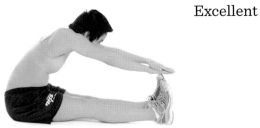

Excellent

Flexibility Score Card

Use a pencil to record your score and check your progress every 4 to 8 weeks.

	LOW	GOOD	EXCELLENT*
	-1	0	+1

Trunk Rotation: _____ Left _____ Right _____

Parallel Squat: _____

Shoulder Mobility: _____ Left _____ Right _____

Back Extension: _____ Left _____ Right _____

Hip Rotation: _____ Left _____ Right _____

Straight Leg Raise: _____ Left _____ Right _____

Sit and Reach: _____

Date _____ Total Score _____   Date _____ Total Score _____

Date _____ Total Score _____   Date _____ Total Score _____

Date _____ Total Score _____   Date _____ Total Score _____

*While excellent flexibility is advantageous, hypermobility may increase your chance for injury.

	LOW	GOOD	EXCELLENT*
	-1	0	+1

Trunk Rotation: _____   Left _____   Right _____

Parallel Squat: _____

Shoulder Mobility: _____   Left _____   Right _____

Back Extension: _____   Left _____   Right _____

Hip Rotation: _____   Left _____   Right _____

Straight Leg Raise: _____   Left _____   Right _____

Sit and Reach: _____

Date _____   Total Score _____   Date _____   Total Score _____

Date _____   Total Score _____   Date _____   Total Score _____

Date _____   Total Score _____   Date _____   Total Score _____

*While excellent flexibility is advantageous, hypermobility may increase your chance for injury.

Stretching Tools and Props

Throughout Part 2 of this book, we'll refer to different stretching tools and props we feel will help you reach your flexibility goals and as add variety to the basic stretches. These are relatively inexpensive and can be found at a local store that carries fitness equipment, or some may even be substituted by items lying around your house.

Foam roller: The foam roller is used to release tension in the muscles, and provides effects similar to receiving a massage. The foam roller can be used on most muscle groups and is a great warm-up tool for any activity.

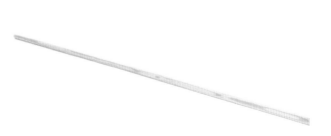

Dowel rod: This could easily be replaced with a broomstick. It often accompanies rotational poses and overhead movements around the shoulders to accomplish a greater range of motion.

Risers: Any sturdy elevated surface can serve the same function as risers for many stretches shown in the book. However, the risers are nice because you can adjust the height to what fits you best.

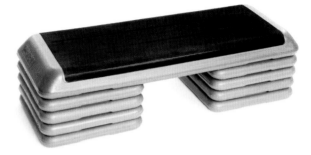

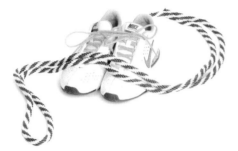

Stretch rope: Simply a rope that can be purchased at any home goods store. This piece of equipment assists a movement and provides a deeper stretch to the targeted muscle group. A 7-foot length works fine.

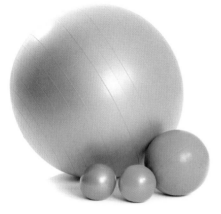

Stability ball and medicine balls: Many different size balls are utilized throughout this book. The large ball is known as a stability ball and can be purchased at many stores that carry fitness equipment. The stability ball adds an extra element to many stretches by incorporating a balance component or a greater range of motion. Medicine balls of various sizes are also used as props, but any type of sport ball will work as well.

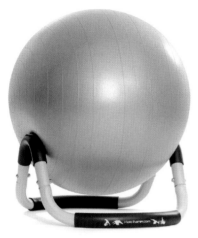

Supported stability ball: Using a support frame, or Halo™, with the stability ball will provide a stationary platform with more stability when needed. This can also be replaced by a sturdy chair for most of the stretches.

Basic Anatomy

A basic understanding of the muscles of the body is important when stretching. Individual stretches will discuss which muscles should benefit from the stretch. If you're unsure where that muscle is located, use the pictures below as a quick reference.

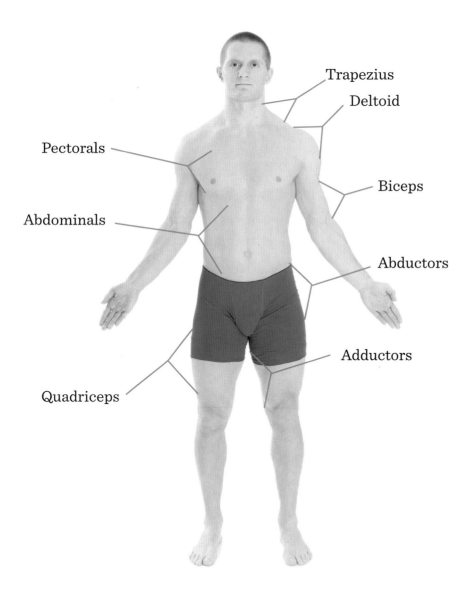

Trapezius

Deltoid

Pectorals

Biceps

Abdominals

Abductors

Adductors

Quadriceps

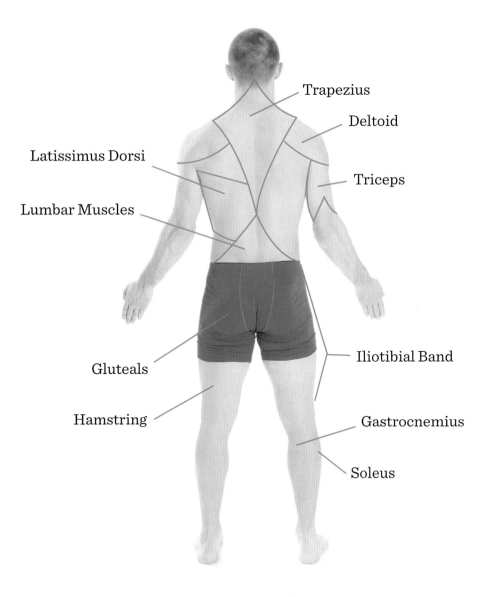

Trapezius

Deltoid

Latissimus Dorsi

Triceps

Lumbar Muscles

Iliotibial Band

Gluteals

Hamstring

Gastrocnemius

Soleus

Part 2

The Stretches

Part 2 includes photos, step-by-step instructions, and modifications for a variety of stretches for each area of the body. The stretches are grouped by parts of the body so it will be easy to find a stretch for a specific muscle. You'll be introduced to a variety of helpful techniques that have a specific place in your flexibility routine, including foam roller exercises, dynamic movements, static stretches, and rope-assisted stretches.

You'll experience the amazing difference in how your muscles feel after something as simple as rolling over a piece of foam. You'll learn that dynamic movements are not just for athletes, and how important it is to train your muscles to work in unison. You'll find plenty of photos, detailed instructions, and useful information for static stretches for every muscle group in the body.

Then you'll go a step further by targeting some muscles using rope stretches to maximize their range of motion. Take notice in this section of the cues on where to feel the stretch, as well as sidebars with helpful tips and both easier and more challenging modifications.

It's up to you to make the time, stretch smart, and stick with it. Your body will reward you, and your other sports and activities will be easier for it.

neck

Neck Extension

It's easy to relax into a forward head tilt when you're sitting at your desk reading a book for a short period of time. If the muscles that extend the neck aren't properly engaged, they may be weak and inflexible. This is a great stretch to counteract this imbalance. You can perform the stretch either seated or standing.

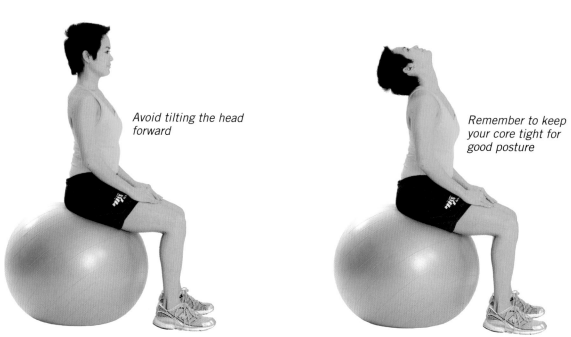

Avoid tilting the head forward

Remember to keep your core tight for good posture

1 Start in a seated position with your feet flat on the floor and hands resting on your thighs, with your neck straight and eyes looking forward.

2 Begin by pulling your chin up toward the ceiling, while keeping your shoulders relaxed. Return to the start position before repeating the stretch.

Neck Flexion

You can gain flexibility of the neck through a variety of stretches. To increase range of motion in a downward direction, use this exercise as a gentle stretch to improve flexion. You can perform this stretch either seated or standing.

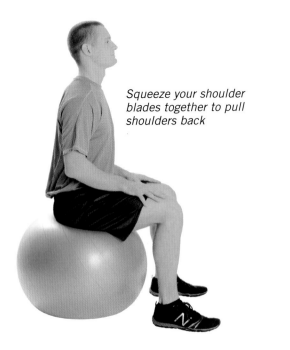

Squeeze your shoulder blades together to pull shoulders back

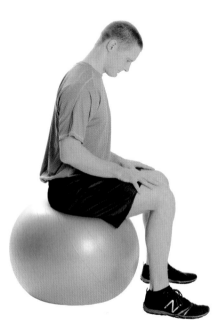

1 Begin in a seated position with your feet flat on the floor and hands resting on your thighs. Start with your neck straight and eyes looking forward.

2 Using your core muscles to keep your back straight for the duration of the stretch, begin the movement by tucking your chin downward toward your chest. Keep your shoulders relaxed. Hold and return to the start position to relax the stretch.

Side Neck Stretch

There aren't many tasks that require us to bend our neck from side to side. Yet the tension from daily stresses gathers in this very area, leaving these muscles tight and with limited range of motion for many people. This gentle stretch helps release tension from the neck.

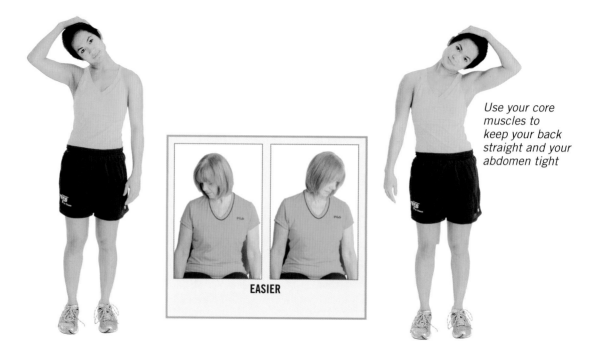

EASIER

Use your core muscles to keep your back straight and your abdomen tight

1 Standing with your feet shoulder width apart and arms relaxed at your sides, start with your neck straight and eyes looking forward. Place your right hand on top of your head and slowly lower your right ear toward your shoulder until you feel the muscles fully lengthen on the left side of the neck.

2 Return to the start position to relax the neck. Then place your left hand on top of your head and repeat the stretch toward the left until you feel the tension on the right side.

Side Neck Rotation

We depend many times during the day on the ability of our neck to rotate freely—to look left and right before turning the car, or to quickly look over our shoulder when we hear something behind us. This stretch helps to improve this range of motion by exaggerating a movement we use so often.

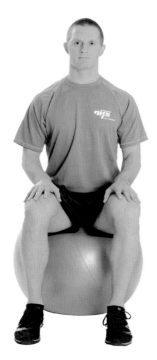

Keep your back straight with your core muscles activated and your chin level

1 Seated with your feet flat on the floor and your hands resting on your thighs, start with your neck straight and tall and your eyes looking forward.

2 Begin the movement by slowly turning your head to the left until you feel tension in the right side of your neck. Return to the start position to relax the neck and repeat the stretch on the right side.

shoulders

Shoulder Circle Progression

Your shoulder has the greatest range of motion of any joint. It's also one of the most often injured, thanks to a complex arrangement of ligaments, tendons, bursa sacs, and bones. To keep this joint mobile, it's critical to stretch your shoulder through its full range of motion every day. This dynamic movement is an excellent way to improve shoulder mobility.

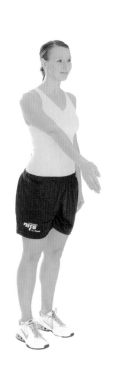
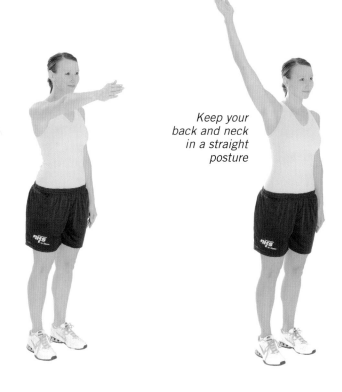

Keep your back and neck in a straight posture

1 Standing with your feet shoulder width apart and your core tightened, start with small circles one arm at a time. Rotate forward 5 circles and backward 5 circles. Switch arms and repeat.

2 Next, make medium-size circles. Rotate forward 5 circles and backward 5 circles, and gradually increase the size of the circle as you go. Switch arms and repeat.

3 For the final flow of the movement, progress to the largest circles possible. Rotate forward and then backward 5 to 10 times in each direction.

Standing Rotator Cuff

Your rotator cuff is a group of muscles and tendons attached to the bones in the shoulder joint. The combination provides stability to the joint while giving the shoulder 360 degrees of motion. This functional warm-up is a good stretch to prepare for strength training or other fitness activities.

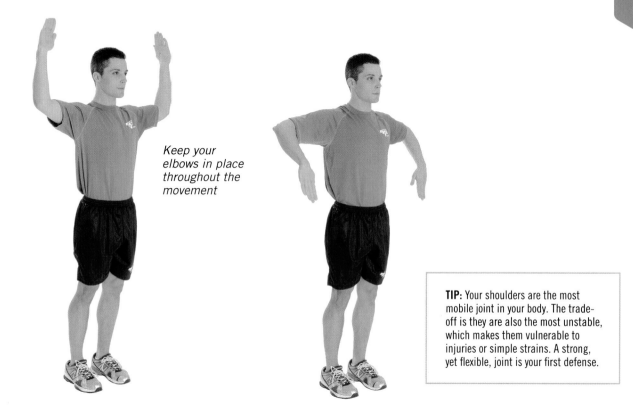

Keep your elbows in place throughout the movement

TIP: Your shoulders are the most mobile joint in your body. The trade-off is they are also the most unstable, which makes them vulnerable to injuries or simple strains. A strong, yet flexible, joint is your first defense.

1 Stand tall with your abdominals drawn in and glutes tight. With your elbows at 90 degrees, position your upper arms parallel to the ground. Your palms are facing forward with fingers pointing to the ceiling.

2 Gradually rotate your arms downward until you feel resistance. Slowly return to the start position until you again feel resistance. Continue using controlled momentum in a pain-free zone for one set of 5 to 10 reps.

Shoulder Roll

When our shoulders become tense, blood flow is slowed to the area. The less blood, the less oxygen. The less oxygen, the more fatigue. The purpose of the shoulder roll is to learn to isolate, mobilize, and ultimately relax the neck and shoulder muscles.

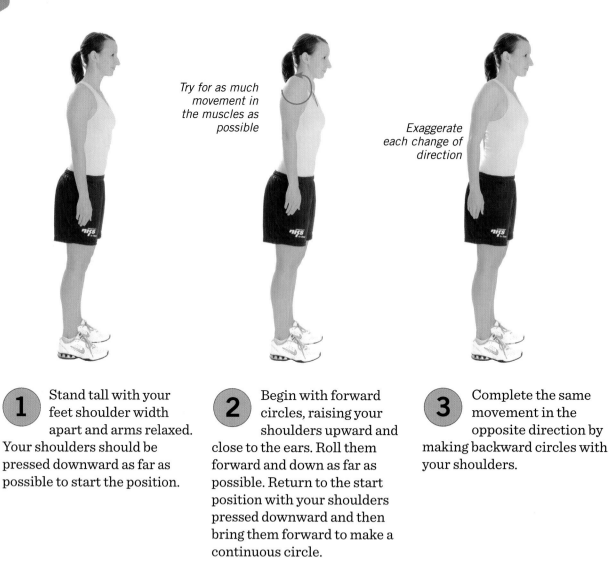

Try for as much movement in the muscles as possible

Exaggerate each change of direction

1 Stand tall with your feet shoulder width apart and arms relaxed. Your shoulders should be pressed downward as far as possible to start the position.

2 Begin with forward circles, raising your shoulders upward and close to the ears. Roll them forward and down as far as possible. Return to the start position with your shoulders pressed downward and then bring them forward to make a continuous circle.

3 Complete the same movement in the opposite direction by making backward circles with your shoulders.

Behind Back Shoulder Reach

Tight chest muscles, often combined with weak upper back muscles, can lead to a forward slouch of the shoulders. This stretch allows the shoulders to retract and the chest to open up to help alleviate the slouching and encourage better posture.

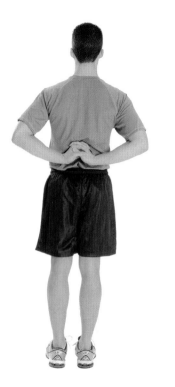

Practice pulling the shoulders back without your hands behind your back

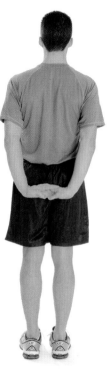

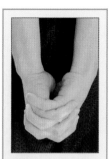

EASIER: Clasp your hands so the palms are facing upward.

 1 Stand with your feet shoulder width apart and arms bent behind your back. Begin with your fingers interlocked behind your back, palms facing downward, and shoulders relaxed.

2 Keeping your fingers interlocked and your back flat, press your shoulders back until you feel the stretch in the chest and front of the shoulders.

Overhead Shoulder Reach

How many times a day do you reach overhead? Chances are it's not many, our surroundings have become so convenient. The more you practice this movement, the easier common tasks like reaching for a high cabinet door become.

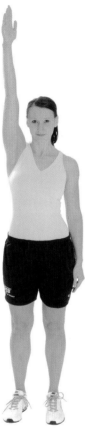

Keep as straight a line as possible from from the arms to the feet

1 Standing with your feet shoulder width apart, reach your right arm straight up toward the ceiling until you feel a stretch in the shoulder along the right side. Then switch arms and reach high with your left arm.

2 For the final movement, reach both arms up over your head toward the ceiling until you feel a stretch on both sides of your body.

Backhand and Forehand Swing

Sports such as golf, tennis, and badminton require excellent shoulder flexibility and strength. Use this dynamic movement as part of an active warm-up. Begin slowly and allow the weight of your arm to gradually increase speed and range of motion.

Track your hand with your eyes while keeping your neck in line with your spine

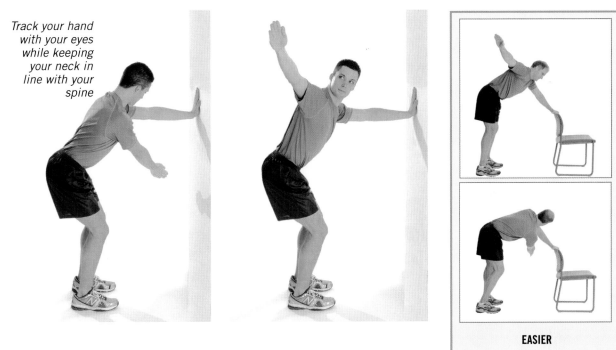

EASIER

1 Place your left hand on a wall and extend the arm fully. Reach your right arm across your chest and under your left shoulder by dropping your right shoulder until you feel the stretch in the back of the shoulder.

2 Complete the backhand by swinging the right arm back through the start position and allowing the momentum to raise the extended arm as high over the right shoulder as possible.

Straight Arm Crossover

It's easy to ignore what we don't see, and this is often the fate of the posterior shoulder muscles. What makes these smaller muscles so significant is the way they work with the upper back muscles to stabilize and move the shoulder blades. The more flexibility and control you have in your shoulders, the more dexterity you have in your hands.

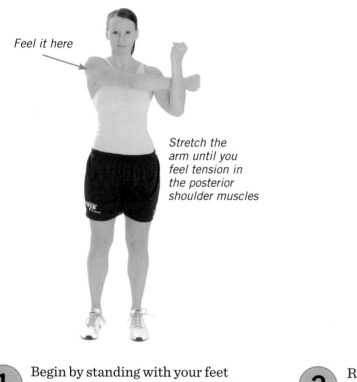

Feel it here

Stretch the arm until you feel tension in the posterior shoulder muscles

Feel it here

1 Begin by standing with your feet shoulder width apart and your right arm extended across the chest. Hook your left arm under the right forearm to hold the right arm in place. Use your left arm to press the right arm inward toward your chest.

2 Repeat the stretch on the opposite side by placing your right arm under the left forearm to hold the left arm across your chest. Using the right arm for assistance, press the left arm inward toward your chest.

Kneeling Reach, Roll, and Lift

It's often the smallest muscles around a joint that limit your range of motion. This exercise does an excellent job of opening up the shoulder joint and activating the hard-to-isolate muscles on the back side of the shoulder.

 Begin on your hands and knees with your head facing the floor. Extend your arms out in front of you, palms on the floor, with your head and neck in a neutral position.

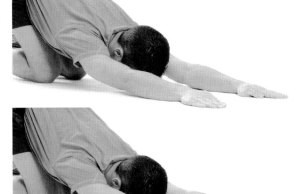

 Keep your left arm in place throughout the movement and your right arm straight out in front of you, turning your right palm up.

 Raise your arm up off the floor as far as you can without straining.

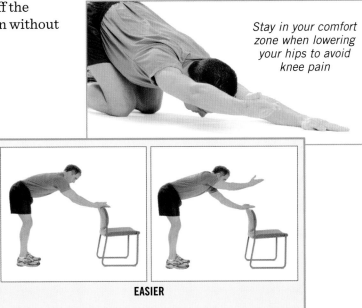

Stay in your comfort zone when lowering your hips to avoid knee pain

EASIER

arms, wrists, and hands

Bent Arm Crossover

The triceps muscle behind the upper arm has three distinct heads. Because each works best from a different angle, it's important to stretch the upper arm in multiple directions. To fully benefit from the Bent Arm Crossover, be careful not to rotate your trunk at the waist.

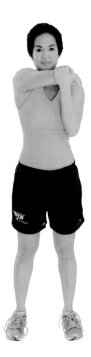

You should feel the stretch in your triceps muscles, but any discomfort is a sign to ease up!

1 Stand with your feet shoulder width apart with your right arm across the chest and bent over your shoulder. With your left arm, pull the right arm across your chest and gently upward until you feel a slight tension in the triceps.

2 Repeat the stretch on the opposite side with your left arm across the chest and bent over your shoulder. Remember to hold your abdominals in and maintain straight posture.

Overhead Triceps Rope Stretch

Our world has become so convenient, it's not often we need to reach overhead or use the full motion of our shoulders and upper arms. This exercise can make reaching for that top shelf in the garage or zipping up a dress much less intimidating.

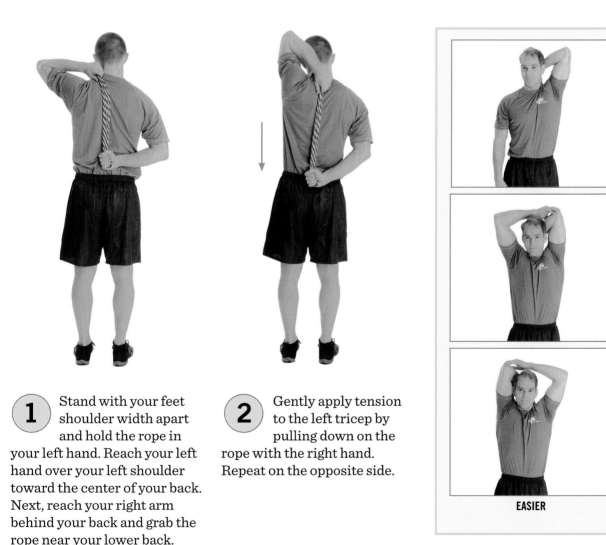

EASIER

1 Stand with your feet shoulder width apart and hold the rope in your left hand. Reach your left hand over your left shoulder toward the center of your back. Next, reach your right arm behind your back and grab the rope near your lower back.

2 Gently apply tension to the left tricep by pulling down on the rope with the right hand. Repeat on the opposite side.

Front Arm Biceps Stretch

The biceps is a difficult muscle to isolate and stretch, so it's often overlooked when exercising. Muscle tears often occur when a sudden heavy effort overstresses a tight biceps, so it's important to keep them in good shape.

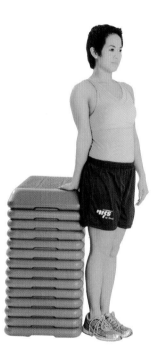 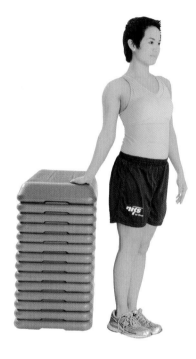

1 Begin the stretch with your right arm straight and reach your right hand backward on a surface that's level with your upper thigh. The rest of your body should be squared and facing forward.

2 Keeping your right hand on the surface behind you and your right arm straight throughout the movement, lean slightly forward. When you feel a gentle stretch in the right biceps muscle, don't lean any farther but hold the pose there.

Wrist Circles

The wrist joint can become an issue when it's overused. Due to the amount of typing many people do during their day, carpal tunnel syndrome has become a common problem. The following movement can alleviate wrist pain by increasing blood flow to the area and can improve overall range of motion.

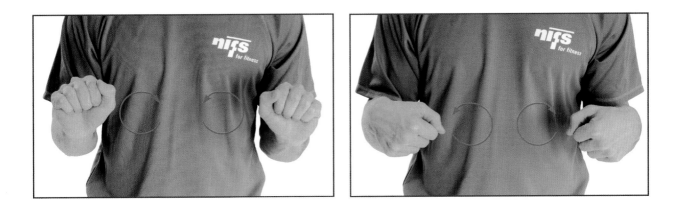

1 Start with your elbows tucked at your sides in a 90-degree angle. Make a gentle fist with each hand. While moving only the wrist joint, slowly circle your fist inward 10 to 15 times.

2 Reverse and circle in the opposite direction 10 to 15 times. Repeat the sequence 2 to 3 times.

Wrist Flexion

Optimal mobility of the wrist joint is key to having good hand dexterity. Writing and unscrewing a lid are two activities we often take for granted that require flexibility in the wrist. This is a quick and easy stretch for any time you wrist feels tight or tired.

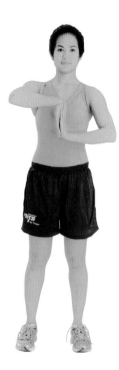 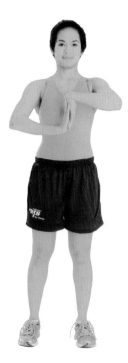

1 Bend your right wrist downward, pointing your fingers toward the floor. Press your left palm against the outside of your right hand. Use your left hand to gently press your right hand down until you feel the tension.

2 Repeat this on the opposite side by bending your left wrist down toward the floor and pressing your right palm against the outside your left hand. Use your right hand to gently press your left hand down until you feel the tension.

Wrist Extension

Most activities require a great deal of wrist flexion, but a lot less extension. This simple stretch improves this often neglected range of motion and can help prevent painful injuries in the future.

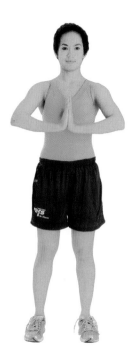
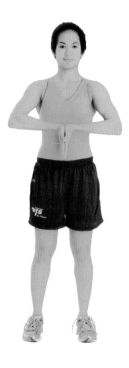

1 Stand straight with your feet shoulder width apart and your shoulders back. Press your palms together in the middle of your chest. Your forearms should be parallel to the floor with elbows out to the side and fingers pointing straight up.

2 Keeping your elbows out to the side and your palms together, rotate your hands away from your body and then downward to complete the stretch. Only rotate your wrists as far as is comfortable and hold for 10 to 15 seconds to complete the stretch. Repeat this movement 5 times.

Finger Flexion and Extension

Repetitive activities (think typing and turning a steering wheel) can quickly lead to fatigue and tightness in your hands. Exercises to extend and flex your fingers are important to avoid overuse injuries and make everyday tasks easier.

Keep your left fingers straight

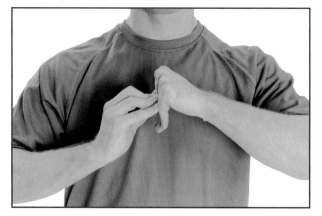

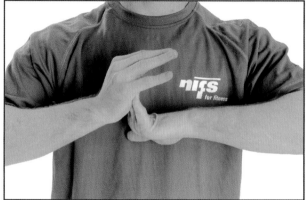

1 Begin by using your right hand to press your left fingers downward and back toward your palm. Press as far as is comfortable until you feel tension in your left fingers. Repeat on the opposite side.

2 Pull the left fingers upward using the right hand to assist the stretch to improve finger extension. Press as far up as is comfortable until you feel tension in your left fingers. Repeat on the opposite side.

chest

Dynamic Chest Movement

Dynamic movements prepare your joints for activity. The repeated muscle stretch and contraction provides a thorough warm-up through a wide range of motion. Golfers and racket sport players will appreciate the feel of this stretch.

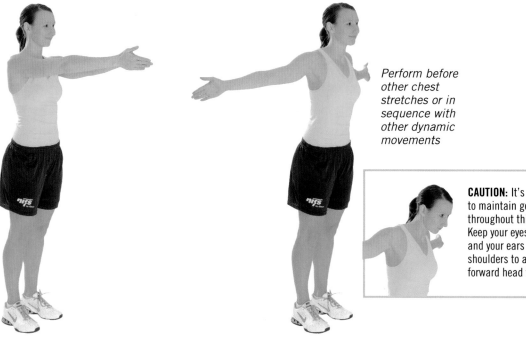

Perform before other chest stretches or in sequence with other dynamic movements

CAUTION: It's important to maintain good posture throughout this exercise. Keep your eyes forward and your ears over your shoulders to avoid a forward head thrust.

1 Start with your feet shoulder width apart and your arms extended in front and parallel to the floor.

2 Keep your arms extended and pull them back as far as possible. Return to the starting position to complete the movement. Repeat 8 to 10 times with a minimal pause between each change of direction.

Standing Wall Chest Stretch

Some types of conditioning, such as weight lifting, can lead to tight chest muscles. The tightness you feel after a set of bench presses or push-ups is best countered with a chest-opening stretch using a wall or other sturdy surface.

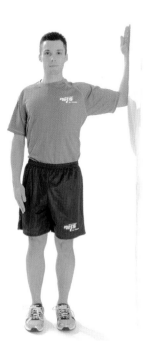

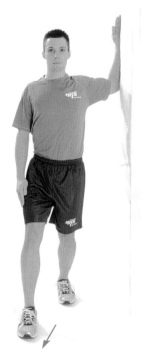

1 Stand with your feet shoulder width apart and your left arm bent at a 90-degree angle. Place the upper part of your left arm against a wall or doorway.

2 Keeping your left arm on the wall, shift your body forward by taking one long step with the right leg. Keep your head up and relax your shoulder, neck, and back muscles. Repeat on opposite side.

Seated Single Arm Chest Stretch

Many people develop a curve in the back and shoulders due to poor posture while sitting at a computer or desk all day. This is an excellent stretch to help correct your desk-job posture without even leaving your desk.

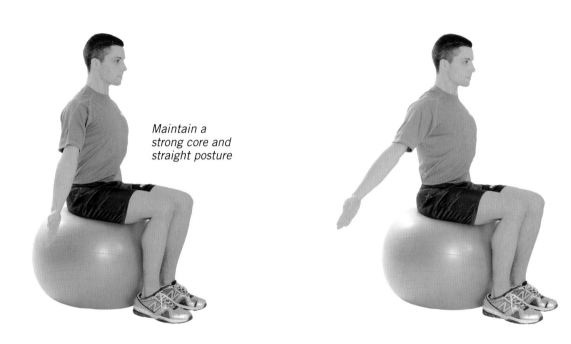

Maintain a strong core and straight posture

1 From a seated position with your feet flat on the floor, extend your right hand toward your right side and press back until you feel a complete stretch in the right side of your chest.

2 Repeat this stretch moving your arm at various angles to feel a stretch in different parts of the chest. Perform 8 to 10 reps and repeat on the opposite side.

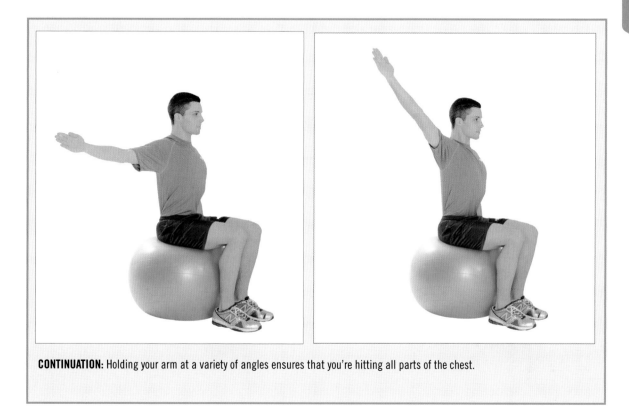

CONTINUATION: Holding your arm at a variety of angles ensures that you're hitting all parts of the chest.

Foam Roller Stretch

The elevated angle of this movement gives a greater range of motion in the shoulders and a deeper stretch in the chest. Get the most out of this relaxing stretch by adding a subtle side-to-side roll.

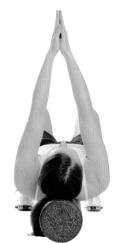

Press the entire length of the spine into the foam roller

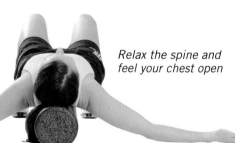

Relax the spine and feel your chest open

1 Lie on your back with your knees bent and feet flat on the ground. Place the foam roller along the spine and extend both arms up over your chest with hands together.

2 Bring both arms down to the ground and straight out to your sides to open up the chest muscles. Hold this stretch for 20 to 30 seconds.

Bent Arm Fly

The longer we stay in one position, whether sitting or standing, the more fatigued our muscle become and the more we compromise our posture. Counteract this tendency with thoughtful activation of the neck and back muscles and stretching movements of the chest.

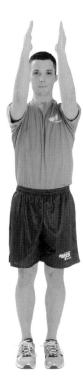 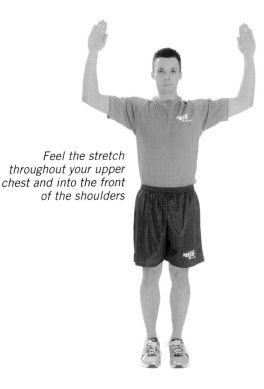

Feel the stretch throughout your upper chest and into the front of the shoulders

1 Stand with your feet shoulder width apart. Keeping your elbows at 90 degrees, hold your upper arms parallel to the floor in line with your shoulders and in front of your chest. Your palms are facing inward and your fingers are pointing to the ceiling.

2 Keeping your arms at 90 degrees throughout the movement, pull your elbows back until you feel a stretch in the chest muscles. Then slowly return to the start position by pulling your elbows back to the front of your body.

TIP: Use the muscles around the shoulder blades to pull your arms back.

Chest Foam Roll

Rolling the chest with the foam roller is a great way to relieve muscle soreness and tightness in this hard-to-reach area. Try this stretch before a weight-lifting workout or the day after to receive the full benefit.

 1 Lie on your stomach with your left arm extended, place the foam roller under the left pec muscle.

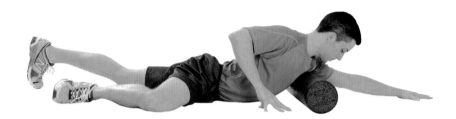

 2 Roll up and down from the mid-torso to below the shoulder. If you feel a spot that's tender or tight, spend more time working that particular area. Roll back and forth for 15 to 30 seconds and then repeat on the opposite side.

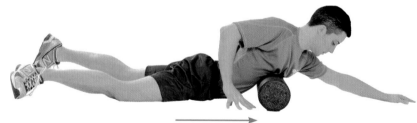

upper
back

Upper Back Foam Roll

Upper back muscles collect a lot of tension throughout the day, and show signs of fatigue by poor posture. Using a foam roller on this area can help to relax the muscles and release the tension.

1 Lie on your back with the foam roller under your upper back, knees bent, and feet flat on the floor. Place your arms behind your head to support the neck. Use your legs to lift your hips off the floor.

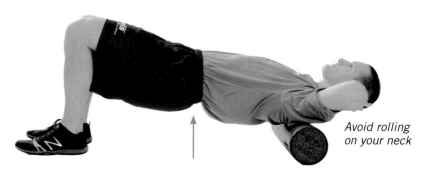

Avoid rolling on your neck

2 Roll up and down your upper back between your shoulders and the bottom of the lat muscles. If you feel a spot that's tender or tight, spend more time working that area. Perform the rolling movement for 15 to 30 seconds.

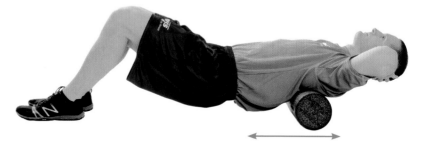

Lats Foam Roll

The latissimus dorsi is the largest muscle in the back. When it feels relaxed, your shoulders and entire back move more freely. If you're looking for a do-it-yourself massage, the foam roller is just the thing.

 1 Lie on your right side with the foam roller under your upper back and extend your right arm overhead.

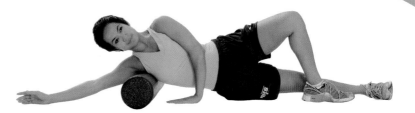

Angle the foam roller so it's resting on the outside of your back.

2 Roll up and down the outer edge of your back. If you feel a spot that's tender or tight, spend more time working that area. Perform the rolling movement for 15 to 30 seconds and then repeat on the left side.

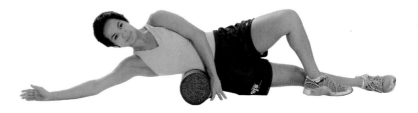

Use the top leg to shift your weight back and forth.

Dynamic Overhead Shoulder Reach

Use this movement to warm up your shoulder and neck muscles before moving on to specific shoulder stretches. You can do this exercise seated or standing. Remember to hold your abdominal muscles strong, back straight, and shoulder blades pulled back.

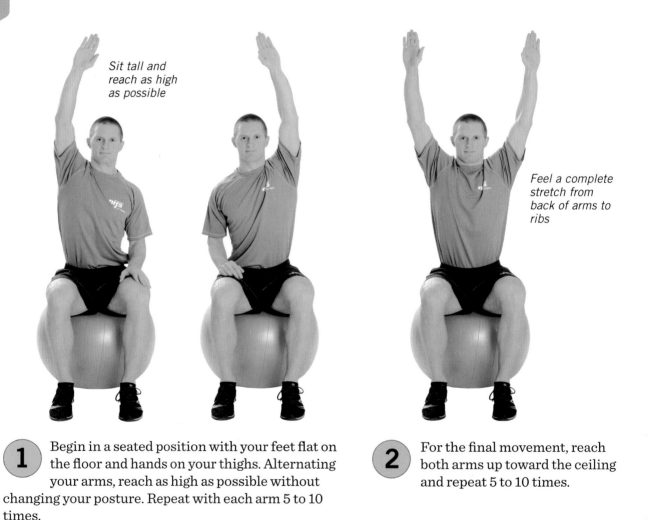

Sit tall and reach as high as possible

Feel a complete stretch from back of arms to ribs

1 Begin in a seated position with your feet flat on the floor and hands on your thighs. Alternating your arms, reach as high as possible without changing your posture. Repeat with each arm 5 to 10 times.

2 For the final movement, reach both arms up toward the ceiling and repeat 5 to 10 times.

Lying Side Reach on Stability Ball

Here's a stretch you don't know you need until you try it. Deeper than a standing overhead reach, the stability ball allows you to completely lengthen the latissimus dorsi from shoulder to low back. The extra stretch you feel in the shoulder and mid-torso shows how these muscles work together

1 Lie on your right side with your torso over the stability ball. Maintain balance with your right hand on the floor and your right leg extended. Bend your left leg over the right for support.

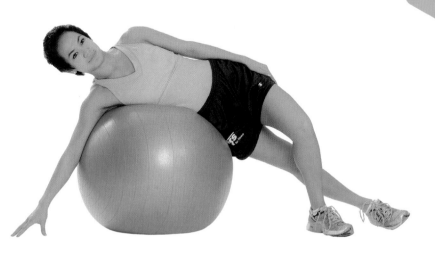

2 Raise your left arm over your head. Reach as far over as possible until you feel a stretch along your left side. Repeat the stretch on the opposite side with your right arm overhead.

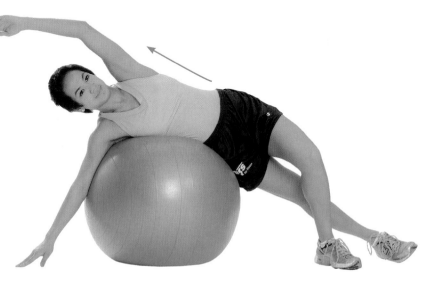

Lat Stretch on Stability Ball

Flexibility in the latissimus muscle is important for good posture. When this muscle is tight it pulls the shoulders forward, separates the shoulder blades, and contributes to "rounded shoulders." This stretch helps to lengthen the muscle.

 Sit up with your knees and toes on the floor and head facing forward. Place both hands on top of the stability ball with your palms up.

> **Modification:** Support the flat back position with one hand on the ground directly under the shoulder and stretch the opposite arm before switching.

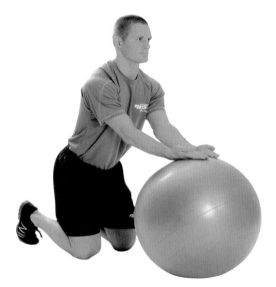

 Slowly roll the ball away from you as you move your upper body into a flat back position. Once you feel slight tension, hold this position for 20 to 30 seconds and return to the start position.

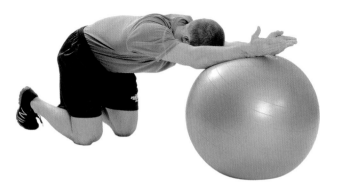

Kneeling One Arm Reach on Stability Ball

Limited range of motion above the head is often due to tight upper back muscles. Releasing the tension in these muscles can improve the ability to perform activities that require reaching above the head. Whether you're serving a tennis ball or reaching for a high shelf, this is an excellent stretch to improve mobility.

 1 From the kneeling position, rotate the hips back to your heels and place your right hand on top of the stability ball in front of you.

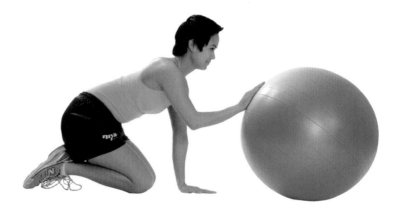

> **TIP:** For an alternative to kneeling, stand with the stability ball against the wall from shoulder height to overhead. Step closer to the wall as your arm reaches higher.

Feel the stretch here

 2 Raise your hips and extend your right arm over the ball until your torso is parallel to the floor and your right arm is fully extended. Feel the stretch along your right side and then repeat with the left arm.

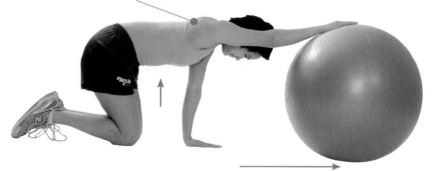

Kneeling Rotation

It's easy to forget how often we depend upon back rotation in daily activities, such as lifting a bag of groceries or throwing a ball. This series of movements isolates the upper back and strengthens the mid-torso and back muscles.

  Begin on your hands and knees with your back level and abdomen tight. Place your right hand behind your head with your elbow pointing straight out.

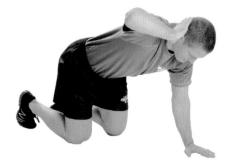

2 Rotate your torso inward, keeping your hand on your head and drawing your right elbow toward your left hand. Turn as far as possible until you feel a complete stretch.

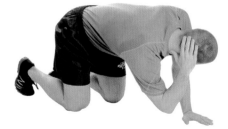

3 To complete the movement, rotate your torso upward as far as possible until you feel the stretch along your left side. Repeat this sequence 3 to 5 times and switch to the left side.

Keep your head and neck in line with your back and open your chest

Child's Pose

Child's Pose is a common yoga move used as a resting pose. Use this pose to release tension in your neck and back with a gentle stretch in the hips, spine, thighs, and ankles. Allow the calming effect of this stretch to relieve stress.

 Start in a flat table top position on your hands and knees. Spread your knees shoulder width apart and keep your big toes touching each other.

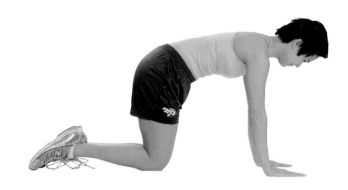

2 Release your shoulders toward the floor, and extend your hands backward to rest by your feet, palms up. Relax in this position for 30 seconds to a few minutes ,taking about 8 deep breaths per minute.

You can stretch your arms out in front with palms down if it's more comfortable

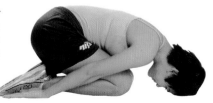

TIP: If you have difficulty sitting back on your heels, place a folded blanket between your thighs and calves.

Extended One Arm Child's Pose

This stretch is a slight variation from the traditional yoga pose. Experiment freely with the arm position until you accomplish a relaxing stretch through the hips, spine, shoulders, and neck.

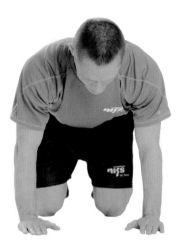

Allow your neck to freely rotate with your shoulder

1 Start in a flat table top position on your hands and knees. Spread your knees slightly wider than you do in the traditional Child's Pose, but still keep your big toes touching.

2 Rotate your hips toward your heels and bring your hands together under your chest. Turn your right shoulder under to reach your hands as far left as you can until you feel the stretch across your upper back. Relax in this position for 30 to 60 seconds, taking 4 to 8 deep breaths, and repeat on the other side.

TIP: For a greater stretch in the hips, thighs, and ankles, lower your hips to your heels.

Kneeling One Arm Lat Stretch

This is similar to but more challenging than Kneeling One Arm Reach on Stability Ball, allowing for a deeper stretch by lowering the body to the floor. Flexible upper back muscles allow for a greater overhead reach and improved range of motion.

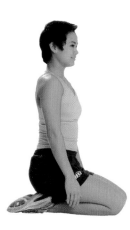

 Begin by sitting upright on your knees and facing forward. Your neck should be in line with the rest of your spine and your arms relaxed at your sides.

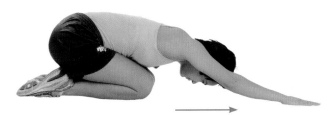

 Gradually lean forward while pressing your hips back toward your heels. Extend your right arm in front as far as possible and your left arm behind, relaxed at your side. Feel the stretch along your right side.

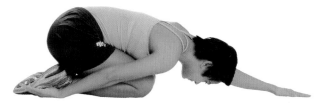

 Repeat on the opposite side by shifting your weight and pressing your hips back toward your heels. Extend your left arm in front and your right arm behind, relaxed at your side.

Half Kneeling Dowel Twist

Torso rotation is essential for sports such as tennis and golf and everyday activities such as driving. These movements isolate the torso from the lower body and improve both internal and external rotation in the upper body.

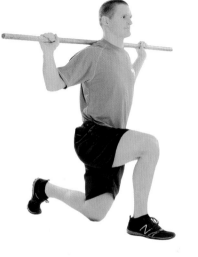 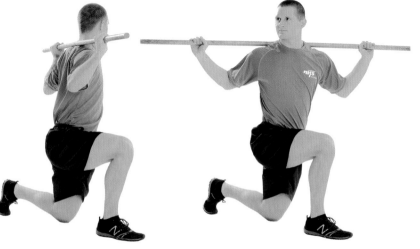

1 Kneeling on the floor with your right foot in front and your left knee on the floor slightly behind, place the dowel across your upper back with one hand on each end. Your core should be tight and shoulders pulled back.

2 Rotate your torso outward over your left knee, keeping the dowel flat across your back. Turn as far as is comfortable until you feel the stretch along your right side. Hold for 10 seconds.

3 To complete the exercise, rotate to the right as far as is comfortable and hold for 10 seconds.

TIP: Maintain straight spinal alignment with your abs tight and shoulders back to get the best benefits from this stretch.

Back Extension on Stability Ball

Whether you sit or stand for long periods of time, a stationary position places a lot of pressure on the spinal column. This explains the discomfort felt after sitting at a desk all day, driving a long distance. This stretch expands and decompresses the spine.

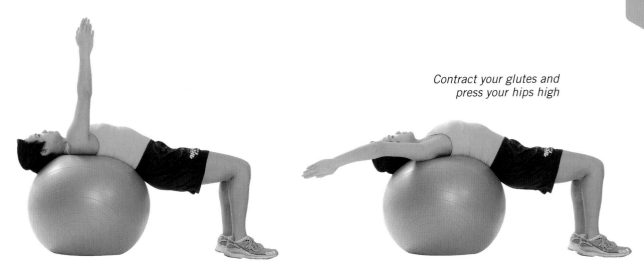

Contract your glutes and press your hips high

1 Begin by lying with your middle to upper back on the stability ball. With your knees bent, plant your feet flat on the floor. Extend your arms above your chest, with hands together and fingers pointed upward.

2 Complete the stretch by reaching your arms overhead. Allow your neck and back to relax. Keeping your arms straight and hands together, gently exhale and inhale as you feel the stretch in the upper back.

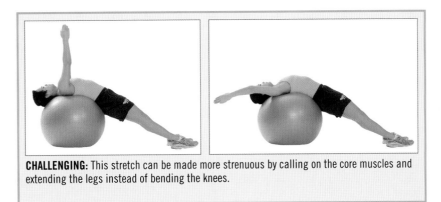

CHALLENGING: This stretch can be made more strenuous by calling on the core muscles and extending the legs instead of bending the knees.

lower
back

Low Back Foam Roll

Lower back pain is one of the leading reasons people visit a doctor or chiropractor. This foam rolling technique releases tension in the lower back, strengthens the muscles, and improves flexibility.

1 Lie on your back with your knees bent and feet on the floor. Place the foam roller in the middle of your back and relax your arms out to the sides.

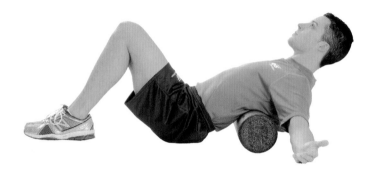

2 Roll up and down the mid- to lower part of your back. If you feel a spot that's tender or tight, spend more time working that particular area. Perform the rolling movement for 15 to 30 seconds.

Cat and Camel

Whether your issue is neck stiffness, low back pain, trouble squatting, or struggling to stand tall, all of these can be improved by increasing flexibility in your spine. This stretch targets the entire length of the spine

1 Begin in a table top position with your back flat, knees on the floor, and hands positioned directly under your shoulders. Your neck should align with your spine.

2 Slowly arch your spine downward by releasing your hips. Press down as far as is comfortable as you exhale.

3 Arch your back upward by rounding your shoulders at the top. Rise up as far as is comfortable as you inhale. Repeat this sequence 5 to 10 times.

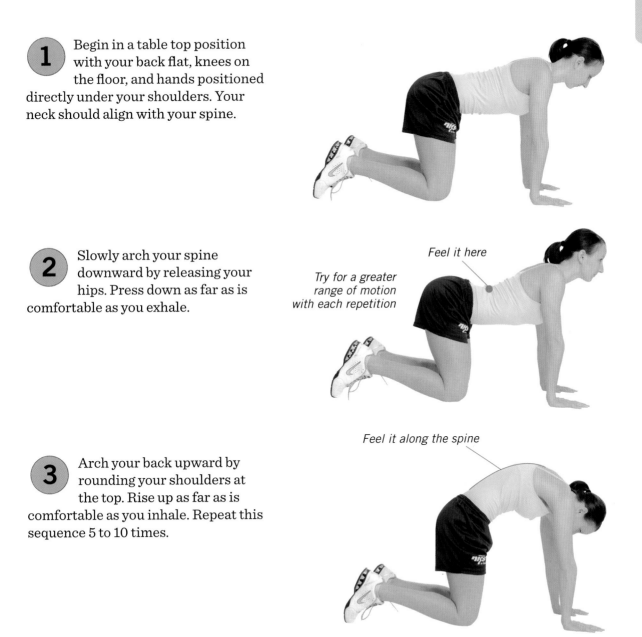

Feel it here

Try for a greater range of motion with each repetition

Feel it along the spine

Spinal Rotation

Low back pain is one of the most common reasons for missed work, but it can be relieved or even prevented with proper stretching. The spinal rotation is great for alleviating low back pain as it allows the spine to elongate and relax, releasing tension and tightness in the area.

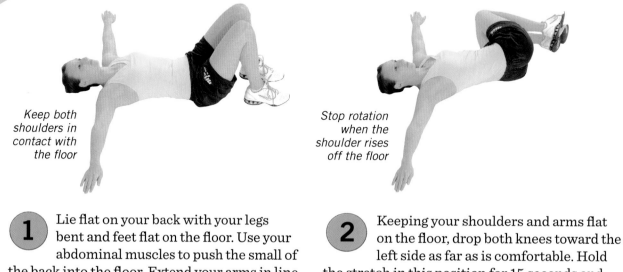

Keep both shoulders in contact with the floor

Stop rotation when the shoulder rises off the floor

1 Lie flat on your back with your legs bent and feet flat on the floor. Use your abdominal muscles to push the small of the back into the floor. Extend your arms in line with your shoulders with palms down.

2 Keeping your shoulders and arms flat on the floor, drop both knees toward the left side as far as is comfortable. Hold the stretch in this position for 15 seconds and repeat on the opposite side.

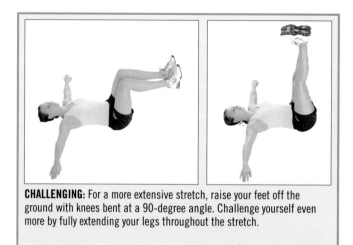

CHALLENGING: For a more extensive stretch, raise your feet off the ground with knees bent at a 90-degree angle. Challenge yourself even more by fully extending your legs throughout the stretch.

Lying Full Body Stretch

Do you find it difficult to get out of bed in the morning because you feel less than fully recharged? This is an excellent stretch to do while lying in bed to get yourself going by waking up your muscles and stimulating your mind.

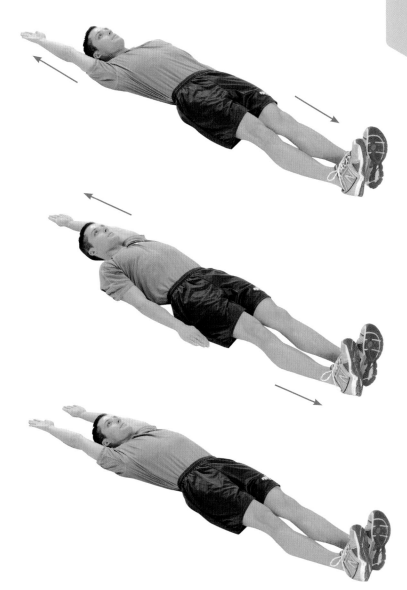

1 Lying flat on your back with your legs together, keep your left arm at your side and reach overhead with your right arm. Push down through your left heel to feel a stretch through your whole body.

2 Next, return your right arm to the start position and repeat the stretch with your left arm overhead. Press down through your right heel.

3 To complete the series, reach as high overhead as you can with both arms and push as far as you can with both heels until you feel a complete stretch.

Stability Ball Reach

Limited mobility in your shoulders can lead to even further limitations throughout your back. This movement activates both shoulder and back muscles to improve flexibility in both areas.

1 Start in a kneeling position with your hands close together on top of the ball and your elbows slightly bent. Keep your core tight and your back flat throughout the movement.

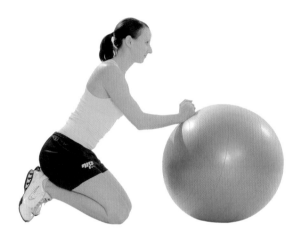

Use a towel or mat to ease pressure on the knees

2 Move your upper body forward slowly to roll the ball out in front of you until you feel a stretch in your upper torso and core. Keep your elbows in contact with the ball for support. Return to the start position by rolling back and shifting your hips back to your heels.

Activate the core muscle to keep your back from arching

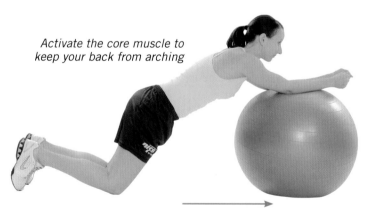

Knee Crossover

Tight hamstrings are often the cause of low back pain. This movement stretches the muscles in the back of the thigh, the buttocks, and the lower back. It helps loosen the hips for improved mobility in the lower back. This stretch makes such tasks easier by giving you more mobility in your lower back.

 1 Start by lying flat on your back with your right arm extended out to the side. Bend your right knee and bring the thigh up to your chest with the assistance of the left arm.

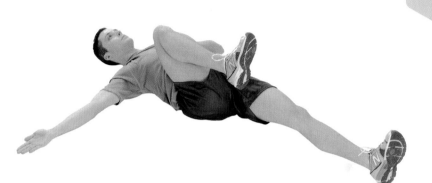

For a greater stretch, use your opposite hand to apply gentle downward pressure above the knee

2 Keeping your shoulders flat on the floor, lower your right leg across your body toward the floor. Turn your head to the right and hold the stretch in a comfortable position for 15 seconds. Repeat on the opposite side.

Single Knee to Chest

Tight hamstrings can restrict movement in the pelvis and lead to back pain and injury. This is one of the most effective stretches for relieving lower back pain, especially when a full leg extension is added.

1 Lie flat on your back with your legs together and arms out to the sides. Point the toes straight up and be sure the small of your back is pressed to the floor.

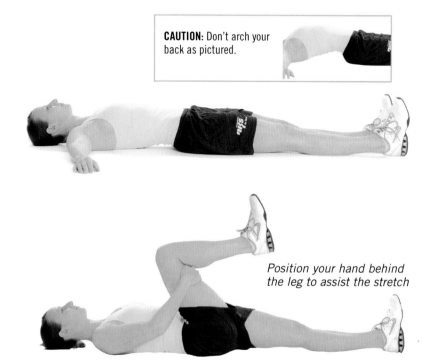

CAUTION: Don't arch your back as pictured.

2 With your right hand, bring your right thigh up to your chest until you feel a stretch in your lower back and hips. Be sure to keep the left leg flat. Hold for 10 to 15 seconds and repeat on the other side.

Position your hand behind the leg to assist the stretch

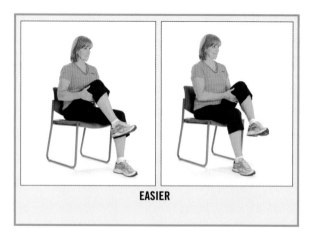

EASIER

Double Knees to Chest

Flexibility of the back muscles and mobility of the spine are important for success in many sports, for both performance and injury prevention. This is a simple stretch that pays a big dividend when it comes to targeting the low back muscles.

 1 Lie flat on your back with your legs together and feet flat on the floor. Be sure that your back is flat and in full contact with the floor.

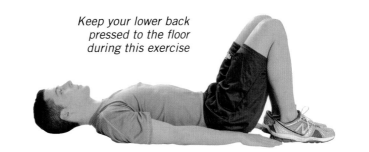

Keep your lower back pressed to the floor during this exercise

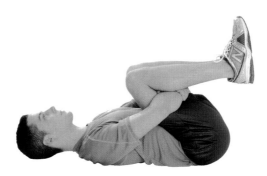 **2** As you lift your legs, lock both arms under your thighs and pull your knees toward your chest. Stop when you feel a stretch to the lower back or if you feel discomfort. Hold the stretch for 15 to 20 seconds.

> **CAUTION:** Do not do this if you feel pain in your low back during the stretch.

> **EASIER:** If you find it too challenging to pull both legs up at the same time, keep one foot flat on the floor as you bring one leg to the chest and then alternate.

Seated Low Back Rotation

Back pain is one of the most common reasons for missed work and visits to the doctor. This pain often results from a lack of physical activity, which leads to weakened muscles. If you have a tight but otherwise healthy back, perform this stretch slowly and gently for an effective mild stretch.

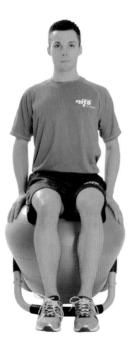

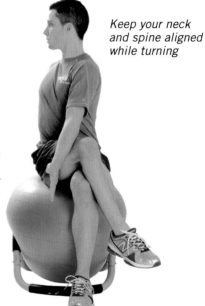

Keep your neck and spine aligned while turning

Apply gentle pressure with your arm against the thigh for a deeper stretch

1 Seated on a stability ball or in a chair with your back straight and core tight, begin with your feet flat on the floor and arms at your sides.

2 Cross your right leg over your left. Turn your torso and shoulders to the right. Hold this position for 10 to 15 seconds and repeat on the opposite side, with the left leg over the right.

Iron Cross

This is an advanced stretch that should be used only by those with no history of back pain. For healthy backs, it's an excellent warm-up to prepare for dynamic movements on several planes. This is important for the rotation needed for everything from gardening to housework to playing basketball.

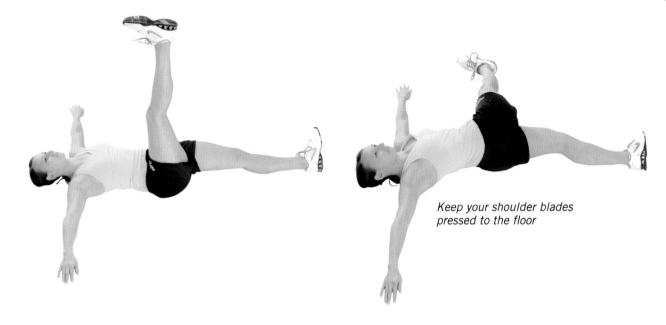

Keep your shoulder blades pressed to the floor

1 Start by lying flat on your back with your arms extended and palms down. Focus on pressing your lower back into the floor. Keep your left leg flat on the floor and lift your right leg straight up.

2 Keeping your shoulders and head flat on the floor, pull your right leg across your body toward the left hand. Lifting only your right hip, reach as far over your body as is comfortable. Hold the stretch for 15 to 20 seconds and alternate between sides 8 to 10 times.

CAUTION: Though this is an easy movement, work at a comfortable pace. Do not do this stretch if you have any back pain or other limiting conditions.

Stability Ball Back Extension

Using the stability ball for this exercise will give you more range of motion than you get on the floor, plus you have the extra challenge of balancing yourself. You'll quickly realize this does more than release tension in your back. Your abs, glutes, and leg muscles all play a role.

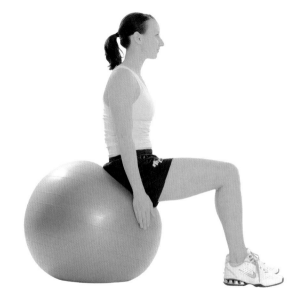

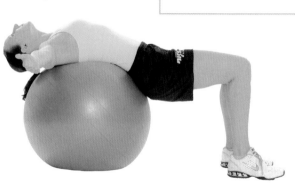

TIP: Prop your feet against the wall for more leverage.

1 Start by sitting toward the front of the stability ball with your arms at your sides and feet flat on the floor. Keep your back straight and core tight while facing forward.

2 Extend your arms out to the sides and roll back onto the ball as you feel a gentle stretch through your back. For a deeper stretch, reach your arms fully overhead and roll back a bit farther. Hold this position for 15 to 20 seconds.

Stability Ball Back Release

With practice, you can train your muscles to relax and let go of the tension that causes tightness and sore muscles. The goal of this stretch is to allow gravity to relax the soft tissue to restore optimal mobility.

1 Start with your feet on the floor, stomach lying over the ball, and knees slightly bent. Place one hand on each side of the ball for balance and support.

Find your balance on the ball before moving into the stretch

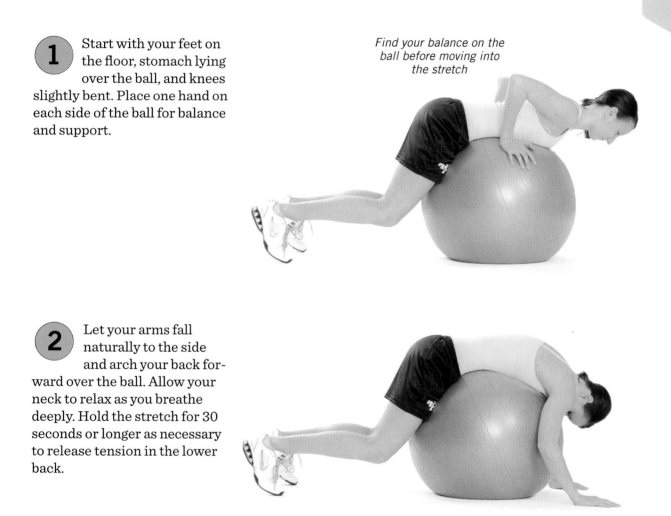

2 Let your arms fall naturally to the side and arch your back forward over the ball. Allow your neck to relax as you breathe deeply. Hold the stretch for 30 seconds or longer as necessary to release tension in the lower back.

core

Core Foam Roll

Core muscles are critical in most daily movements, and therefore are often overused and tight. Since the core muscles don't bear weight, their limitations and tightness often go unnoticed. Use the foam roller to alleviate tension in the outer muscles of the core.

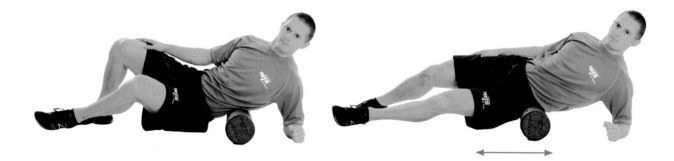

1 Lie on your left side with the foam roller under your mid-torso. Place your left arm on the floor to prop up your upper body, and stack your legs right over left with knees slightly bent to support the lower body.

2 Roll up and down your side between the mid-torso and hips. If you feel a spot that's tender or tight, spend more time working that area. Perform the rolling movement for 15 to 30 seconds and repeat on the opposite side.

Standing Half Moon

Flexibility of the spine is important for good posture and mobility. This modified yoga pose improves the lateral flexibility of the spine, but also warms up all the muscles of the core.

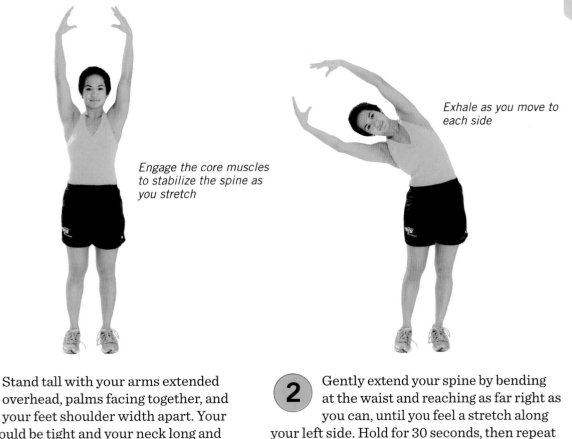

Engage the core muscles to stabilize the spine as you stretch

Exhale as you move to each side

1 Stand tall with your arms extended overhead, palms facing together, and your feet shoulder width apart. Your core should be tight and your neck long and even.

2 Gently extend your spine by bending at the waist and reaching as far right as you can, until you feel a stretch along your left side. Hold for 30 seconds, then repeat on the left side.

> **TIP:** If you sit in a chair all day, try a seated half moon pose to relieve tightness in your lower back and shoulders.

Quad Rock

Tight quadriceps and hip flexors can lead to nagging injuries. The quad rock can increase the flexibility of these muscles by actively increasing their length throughout the movement.

1 Begin the stretch in a flat table top position with both your hands and knees shoulder width apart and your back flat.

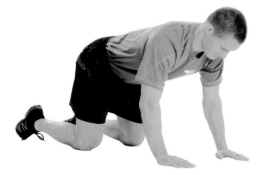

2 Rock your hips back toward your heels while extending your arms out in front. Reach back with your hips as far as possible.

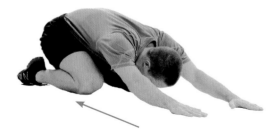

Focus on opening up the front hip area as you rock forward

3 Return to the start position and rock your hips forward until your shoulders are slightly in front of your hands. Feel the stretch along the abdomen, quadriceps, and hip flexors.

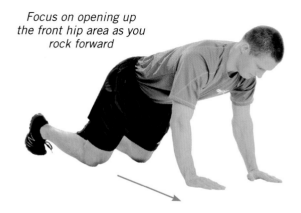

Forward Lunge with Open Torso

Oblique flexibility is important for good posture and back function. When your obliques aren't active, more stress is placed on the lower back. This stretch lengthens the oblique muscle and improves flexibility.

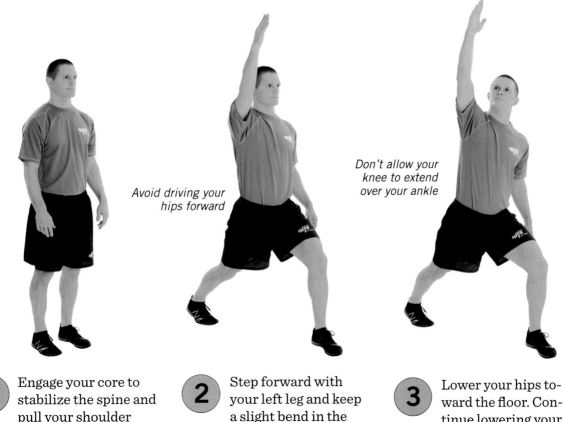

Avoid driving your hips forward

Don't allow your knee to extend over your ankle

1 Engage your core to stabilize the spine and pull your shoulder blades together.

2 Step forward with your left leg and keep a slight bend in the right knee behind you. Slowly shift your body weight onto the front foot and find your balance without wobbling. Raise your right arm high overhead.

3 Lower your hips toward the floor. Continue lowering your body to a comfortable position, or until your thigh becomes parallel to the floor. Return to the start position by firmly pressing off with the front leg. Repeat on the opposite side.

Triangle Pose

This basic yoga pose builds strength, stability, and balance. Don't be intimidated by the degree of movement—it's best approached as an ongoing experiment. Focus your mind on the steadiness of the feet and legs, the expansion of the torso, and the evenness of the arms and legs.

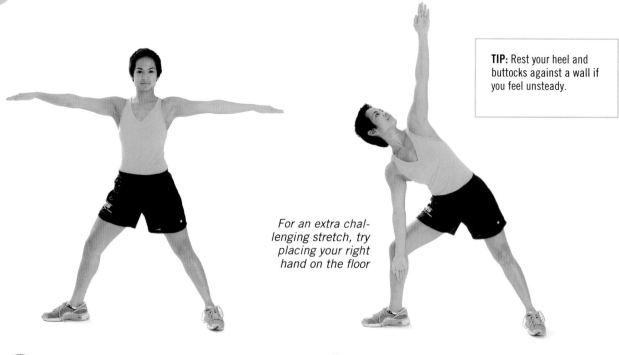

TIP: Rest your heel and buttocks against a wall if you feel unsteady.

For an extra challenging stretch, try placing your right hand on the floor

1 Begin with your feet about 3 feet apart. Turn your left foot in slightly to the right and your right foot out 90 degrees. Keep the center of the right kneecap in line with the right ankle. Raise your arms parallel to the floor, shoulder wide, palms down.

2 Exhale and extend your torso to the right directly over the leg, bending from the hip joint, not the waist. Rest your right hand on your shin or ankle. Stretch your left arm toward the ceiling and let your eyes follow the left hand. Stay in this pose for 30 to 60 seconds and repeat on the opposite side.

EASIER: Use a block or stack of blocks along the outside of your foot for a more comfortable bend at the waist.

Side Overhead Reach on Stability Ball

The stability ball not only adds a balance component to this stretch, it allows you to create a greater angle along the entire side of the body you're stretching. Use the stretch to add a bit of a challenge to your flexibility routine.

TIP: If your balancing arm doesn't reach the floor comfortably, bend your elbow and hold on to the side of the ball.

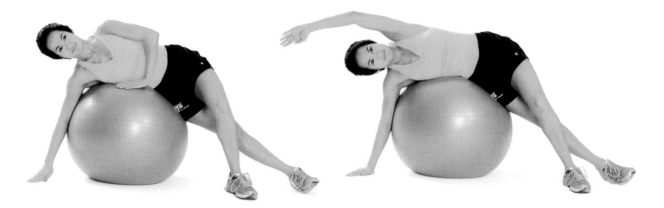

1 Lying on your right side on a stability ball, place your right hand on the floor beside the ball. Reach your right leg behind your torso with the outside of the foot on the ground. Cross your left leg over your right, and with a bent knee, place your left foot flat on the floor.

2 To move into the full position, reach your left arm up over your head. Straighten your left leg out and reach upward to feel the stretch along the left side of your torso. Hold for 20 to 30 seconds and repeat 3 times before switching sides.

Kneeling Thread the Needle

As daily stressors build up, we often don't notice the tension in our upper back until we have a stiff neck or headache. This stretch helps to alleviate the tension by loosening the muscles of the back and neck.

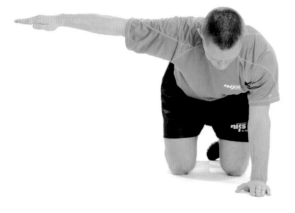 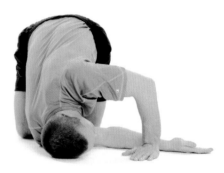

1 Begin the stretch in a flat table top position on your hands and knees. Extend your right arm out to the side in line with your shoulder.

2 To get into the proper stretch position, bend your left elbow down as you reach your right arm along the floor under and across your body. Reach as far as you can until you feel a stretch along the right side or until your right shoulder is on the floor.

EASIER: As an option to getting on the floor for this stretch, try leaning over a table or desk.

Lying Chest Lift (Cobra)

If you're looking for a stretch that's relaxing yet works the entire torso, this stretch is for you! It provides an excellent release for the spine and benefits the abdominal muscles as well as many other muscles and joints.

 1 Begin by lying flat on the floor with your hands shoulder width apart in line with your eyes. Keep your toes on the floor.

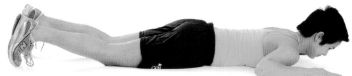

2 Keeping your lower body in contact with the floor, raise your shoulders and head as far as your flexibility allows.

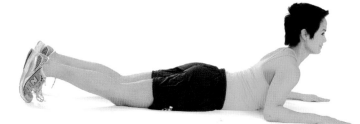

Keep your head in line with your shoulders

3 Extend your arms fully and push your upper body up toward the ceiling, finishing with your neck long and head high.

Feel the stretch throughout your torso

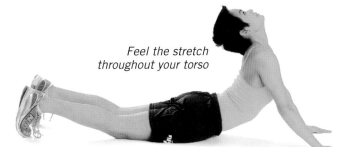

hips

Glute and Piriformis Foam Roll

Foam rolling helps you make the best use of your time by massaging muscles, improving flexibility, and preventing injury. The muscles of the glutes and piriformis can greatly benefit from this combination, as they're used frequently throughout the day.

1 Sit with your left leg slightly bent in front of you and your foot on the floor. Cross your right leg over with your right foot resting on your upper left leg, and place the foam roller under your hips. Put your hands on the floor behind you to prop up your upper body.

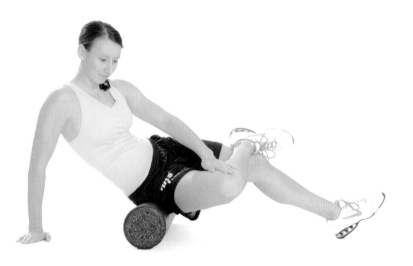

2 Roll up and down the right side of the hips and buttocks. If you feel a spot that's tender or tight, spend more time working that particular area. Perform the rolling movement for 15 to 30 seconds and repeat on the opposite side.

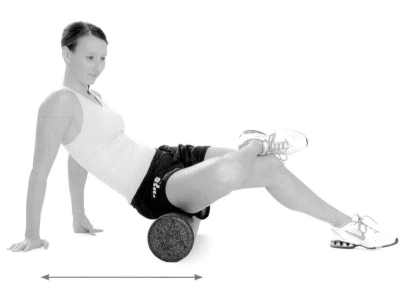

Hip Flexor Foam Roll

Targeting the hip flexor muscles utilizing the foam roller is a great way to alleviate tightness and help prevent injury. These muscles are often hard to isolate when strengthening and stretching, but are used readily throughout the day.

1 Lie on your left side with your left leg extended on the floor and your right leg crossed over. Place the foam roller under your outer left hip. Keep your arms in front of you to prop your upper body up off the floor

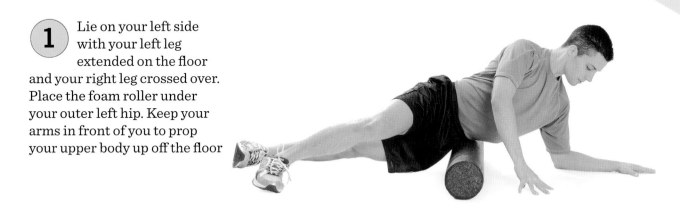

2 Roll up and down the front and outer part of the left hip. If you feel a spot that's tender or tight, spend more time working that area. Perform the rolling movement for 15 to 30 seconds and repeat on the opposite side.

Straighten the legs and hips as you roll upward

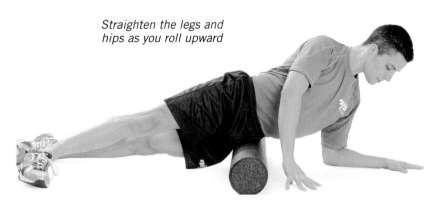

Lateral Leg Swing

Many sports require the ability to complete quick lateral moves for success. Use this dynamic stretch to warm up the hip muscles that perform these moves to maximize performance and minimize injury.

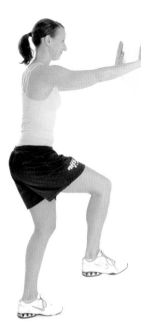 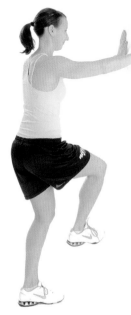

Stand tall for the duration of the sequence to reinforce good posture

1 Lean into a wall or sturdy object for support. Keep your core engaged and back straight. Put your weight on the back leg with a slight bend in the knee. Draw in your abs and raise your right leg.

2 Keeping a bend at the right knee, swing your right leg inward at the hip.

3 Then bring the knee outward across your body, and back to the start position in a continuous sequence. Do this 8 to 12 times, and then repeat using the other leg.

Lateral Lunge

Chances are, you don't have to move side to side very often. This can leave you at risk of losing your balance, and even more susceptible to injury. This dynamic stretch not only increases range of motion in the hips and groin, it also improves lower body strength, balance, and coordination.

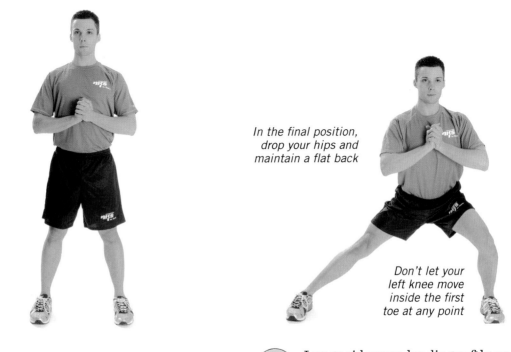

In the final position, drop your hips and maintain a flat back

Don't let your left knee move inside the first toe at any point

1 Stand with your feet shoulder width apart and hands together or on your hips. Keep your core engaged and maintain good posture throughout the movement.

2 Lunge sideways, landing softly on the heel of your left foot with your toes out slightly. Keep your knee in line with your first toes. The lunge knee should be around 90 degrees and the stationary leg should be straight with the knee slightly bent and foot pointing straight ahead. Rise back to the starting position and repeat on the opposite side. Alternate for 5 to 8 reps on each side.

Reverse 90/90

Loosening the muscles of the hips is one way to relieve the symptoms of lower back pain. You get a big bang for your buck with the Reverse 90/90. You may feel a tight IT band along the outside of your thigh as the stretch goes around the hip and into your lower back.

1 Lie flat on your back with your arms fully extended. Bend your right knee and place your right foot on the floor. Cross your left leg over to rest on your right thigh.

2 Keeping your shoulders, upper back, and arms flat on the floor, drop both knees toward the right side. Feel the stretch through your lower back and left hip. Reverse your leg positions and repeat in the opposite direction.

Feel it here

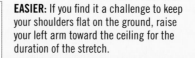

EASIER: If you find it a challenge to keep your shoulders flat on the ground, raise your left arm toward the ceiling for the duration of the stretch.

Standing Outer Hip Stretch

Repetitive movements such as running and biking can lead to tight hip muscles. Opening tight hips is key to alleviating pain associated with the IT band and low back. Use this stretch frequently to open up the hips and keep them loose.

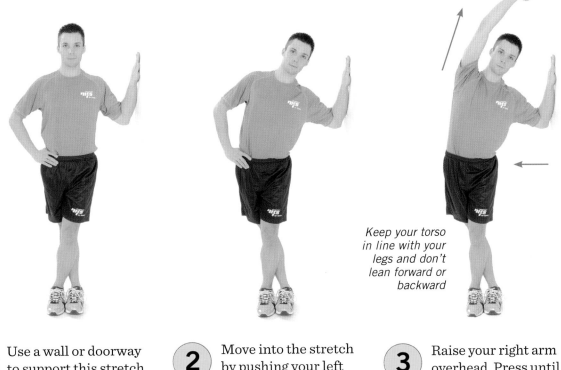

Keep your torso in line with your legs and don't lean forward or backward

1 Use a wall or doorway to support this stretch. With your left side to the wall, place your hand on the wall with a bend in the arm and rest your right hand on your hip. Cross your right leg over your left.

2 Move into the stretch by pushing your left hip away from the wall.

3 Raise your right arm overhead. Press until you feel a stretch throughout the outer right hip. Hold for 15 to 20 seconds and repeat on the opposite side.

Forward Lunge Forearm to Instep

It's very important to keep the hips flexible and strong, as they take considerable stress from everyday activities like walking and climbing stairs. This lunge goes beyond the usual range of motion to open the hip joints and provide a deep stretch in the hips and thighs.

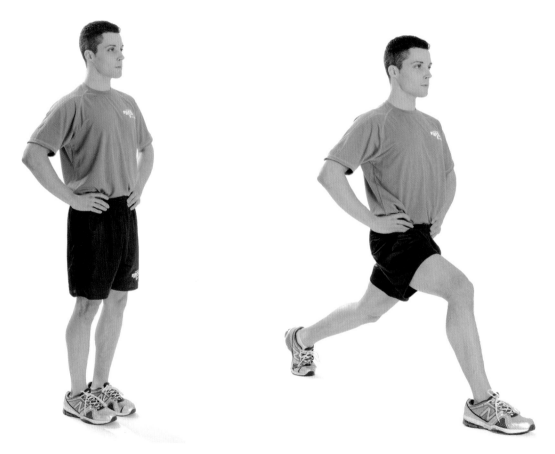

1 Standing tall with your feet shoulder width apart, step your left leg forward with a longer than normal stride. Land softly with weight evenly distributed over the heel and mid-foot, extending your right leg behind.

2 Move into a deep lunge by lowering your hips to the floor, bending your right knee, and placing your left hand on the floor for support.

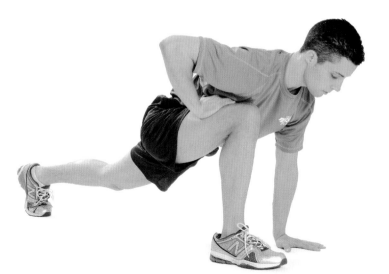

3 Move your right forearm inside the left leg to stretch deeper. Keep your back straight and hold for 15 to 20 seconds, and then repeat on the opposite side.

Feel the stretch through both sides of the hips

Front view

Don't allow your knee to cross over your ankle as you bend the front leg

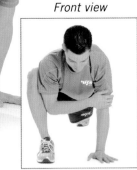

TIP: For more strength and better balance, contract your glutes on both sides throughout this movement. As an added bonus, you'll train your glutes to be engaged in other everyday movements.

Forward Lunge Forearm to Instep

Forward Lunge with Overhead Reach

Performing stretches that combine multiple muscle groups can be very effective. Not only does this allow you to multi-task as far as stretching is concerned, it's also practical because most activities involve more than one major muscle group.

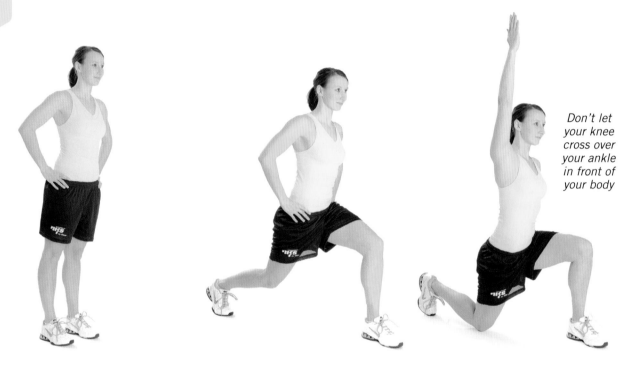

Don't let your knee cross over your ankle in front of your body

1 Stand with your back straight, with feet and legs aligned and hands on hips. Engage your core muscles as you move into the lunge

2 Step forward 3 or 4 feet with your left leg. Keep a slight bend in your right knee back behind you. Slowly shift your weight onto the front foot and find a balance without wobbling.

3 Keeping your torso squared, raise your right arm overhead and drop your hips slightly lower to the floor until you feel the stretch throughout your body. Hold for 15 to 20 seconds. Repeat on the opposite side with your right leg in front, left leg behind, and left arm overhead.

Standing Hip Flexor Stretch

Your hip flexors are a group of muscles responsible for raising your knee to your chest and moving your leg from front to back and side to side. Tight hip flexors are a common cause of low back pain due to their anterior pull on the pelvis. You may want to find more than one hip flexor stretch to work this area from several angles.

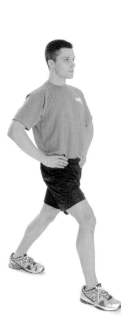 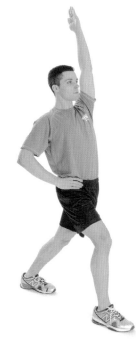

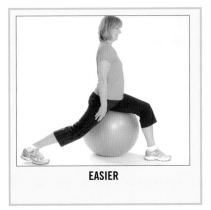

EASIER

1 Stand with your feet staggered, your right leg forward and left leg behind, and both knees bent. Place your hands on your hips, and keep your torso tall and shoulders squared.

2 Move into the stretch by gently lowering your right knee, and raise your left arm overhead. Put most of your weight on the front leg and open the back hip until you feel tension in the left thigh and right hip. Hold for 15 to 20 seconds and repeat on the opposite side.

This is a simple stretch that can be performed almost anywhere, any time you're feeling tight.

Seated Leg Crossover

The hip muscles are vital to keeping your pelvis and low back strong, flexible, and properly aligned. Weak or tight hip muscles can place more work on the back and lead to pain and injury. Master this basic stretch to build strong muscles in the hips and buttocks.

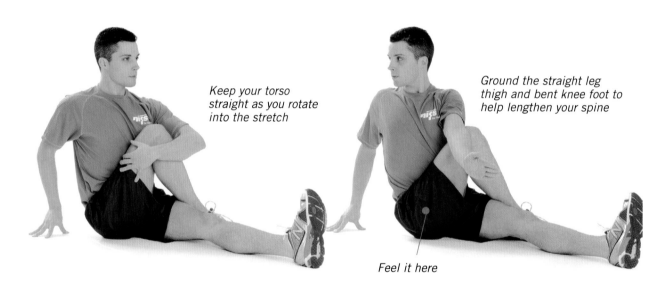

Keep your torso straight as you rotate into the stretch

Ground the straight leg thigh and bent knee foot to help lengthen your spine

Feel it here

1 Sit with your left leg extended out in front and your right leg crossed over. Use your left arm to support the right leg. Keep your back tall, spine aligned, and core engaged.

2 With an exhalation, rotate your torso to the right. Press your right thigh toward your chest and feel the stretch in the outer right hip. Lengthen the spine on the inhalation and rotate slightly more with each exhalation. Hold for 20 to 30 seconds and repeat on the opposite side.

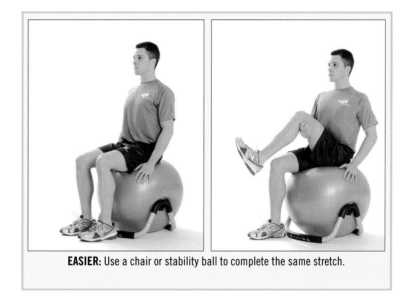

EASIER: Use a chair or stability ball to complete the same stretch.

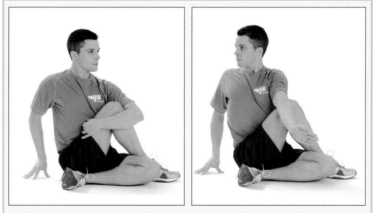

CHALLENGING: For a deeper stretch in the entire hip, bend the extended leg back so your ankle is under your buttocks.

Standing Piriformis Stretch

A tight piriformis can lead to pain in the lower back, buttocks, and leg. This can be caused by overdoing an activity such as running, or even sitting for an extended time. This stretch can be performed on a table or riser that's close to the height of your hip. Try several positions until you find the one that's best for you.

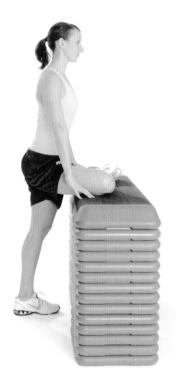 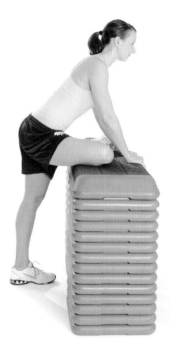

1 Lay your right leg as flat as possible on the riser, bending inward so your foot is pointed to the left. Your right knee should be in line with the foot and your hands rest on the riser.

2 Keeping your core tight and back flat, slowly bend forward at the hips. Move as far forward as is comfortable until you feel the stretch in the hips and buttocks. Hold for 15 to 20 seconds.

This stretch is most effective in a contract/relax sequence

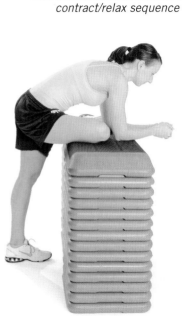

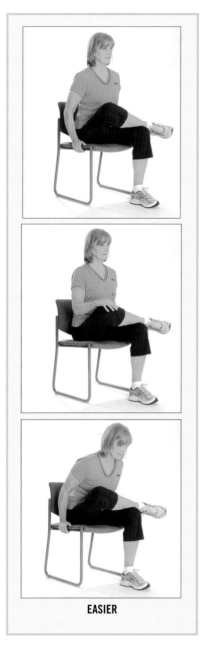

EASIER

 3 Contract your outer hip muscles by pressing the knee down toward the surface for 5 seconds relax and move further into the stretch. Repeat 2 or 3 times and switch legs.

Advanced Piriformis Stretch

An excellent stretch for the entire body, this pose especially targets the hips and piriformis muscle but is only for those who have sufficient flexibility. When performed properly, this stretch can help prevent injury and relieve pain through increased range of motion.

CAUTION: This stretch is not for anyone who has knee or back problems.

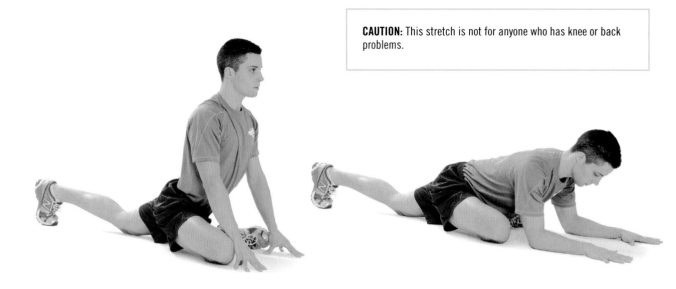

1 Keeping your torso upright, extend your left leg behind and bend your right leg inward across the front of your body.

2 Lower your torso to the floor until you feel the stretch in the hips and glutes. Keep your lower body in the start position with your arms out in front for support. Hold the stretch for 20 to 30 seconds and repeat on the opposite side.

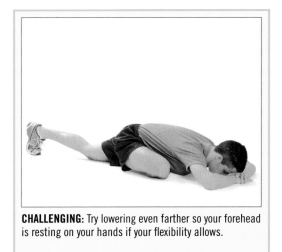

CHALLENGING: Try lowering even farther so your forehead is resting on your hands if your flexibility allows.

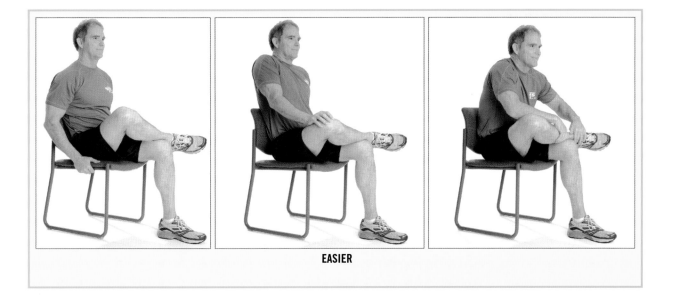

EASIER

Advanced Piriformis Stretch   123

IT Band and Glute Rope Stretch

If you're prone to IT band syndrome or runner's knee, this is a good stretch for you. When this band gets tight, bad things can happen to your gait, not to mention a lot of pain and suffering.

Note that the rope comes off the outside of the foot and under the calf to position the foot with an outward rotation

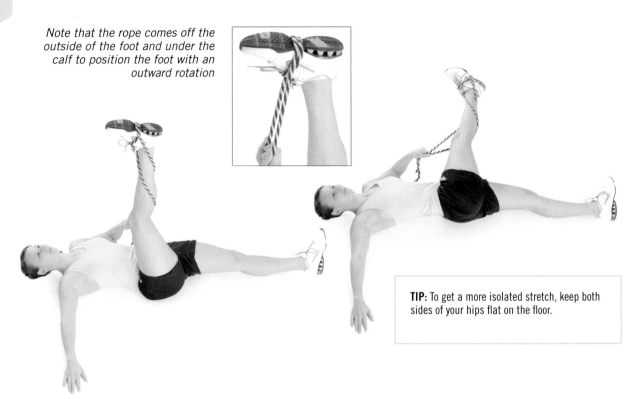

TIP: To get a more isolated stretch, keep both sides of your hips flat on the floor.

1 Lie on your back with both legs extended and the rope wrapped around the midsole of your right foot. Hold both sides of the rope in your left hand, and extend your right arm to the side.

2 Keeping your right leg extended, pull the rope to the left side to bring the right leg across the body until you feel a stretch in the outer leg. Your right arm and left leg shouldn't leave the floor. Hold for 15 to 20 seconds and repeat on the opposite side.

Adductor Rope Stretch

The hip adductors play a big role in everyday movements such as walking and sitting down. They provide stability to the hip joint, allowing better performance in physical activities. Having good range of motion in these muscles is critical for an active lifestyle.

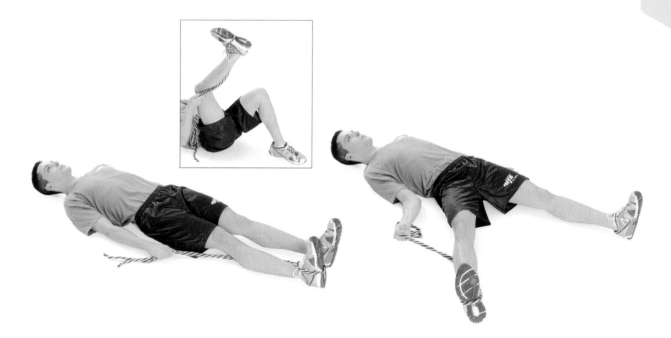

1 Lie fully extended on your back with the rope around the middle of the right foot. Take both ends of the rope over the inside of the ankle and wrap it around to the outside of the calf.

2 Hold both ends of the rope in your right hand. Pull out to the right as far as is comfortable, feeling the stretch along the inside of the right leg. Hold for 15 to 20 seconds and repeat on the opposite side.

upper legs

IT Band Foam Roll

IT band tightness is a common complaint among runners and cyclists. It can often be prevented by properly stretching and warming up the muscles of the upper leg before running. Using the foam roller before and after a run can help you avoid this condition and keep you going pain free!

1 Lie on your side with the foam roller under the outside of your upper right leg. Rest your right arm on the ground to prop up your upper body and bend your left leg over your right to support the lower body.

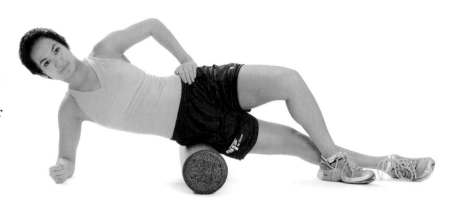

2 Roll up and down the outside of your upper leg between the hip and knee. If you feel a spot that's tender or tight, spend more time working that area. Perform the rolling movement for 15 to 30 seconds and repeat on the opposite side.

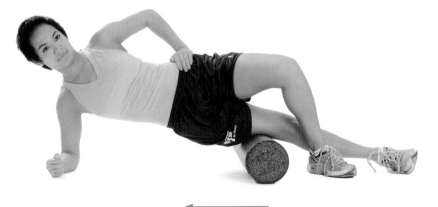

Adductor Foam Roll

The adductor muscles are commonly overlooked. The muscles are constantly in use but are often forgotten when doing other strengthening exercises and stretches. Using a foam roller on this muscle group can help keep them flexible and free from injury.

Don't roll directly on the knee joint

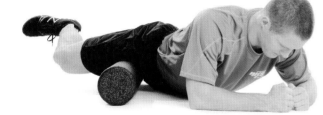

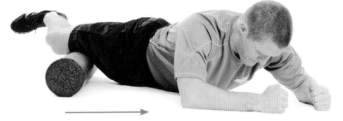

1 Lie on your stomach with the foam roller under your upper right leg. Turn your right foot outward so the foam roller is on the inside of the leg. Place your arms on the floor in front of you to prop up your upper body, and keep your left leg on the ground to support the lower body.

2 Roll up and down the inner part of the upper right leg between the hip and knee. If you feel a spot that's tender or tight, spend more time working that area. Perform the rolling movement for 15 to 30 seconds and repeat on the other leg.

Quadriceps Foam Roll

The quadriceps are a large, frequently used muscle group, so it's hard to ignore them when they're tight and sore. The tightness can lead to low back and hip pain as well. Using a foam roller to release tension and lengthen the muscle can help alleviate these problems.

1 Lie on your stomach with the foam roller under your upper legs. Rest your arms on the floor in front of you to prop up your upper body, and keep your toes on the floor to support your lower body.

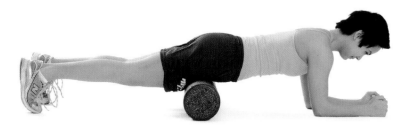

2 Roll up and down the upper leg between the hip and knee, applying just enough pressure to feel the effects of the roller. If you feel a spot that's tender or tight, spend more time working that area. Roll for 15 to 30 seconds and repeat on the other side.

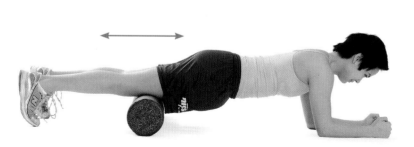

CHALLENGING: Stack one leg over the other to isolate and roll one leg at a time with more pressure applied.

Hamstring Foam Roll

Often weak and overworked, the hamstrings are prone to tightness and injury. For many people the quads are stronger than the hamstrings, and this leads to muscle imbalances and injuries. Use the foam roller to strengthen your hamstrings and help prevent injury.

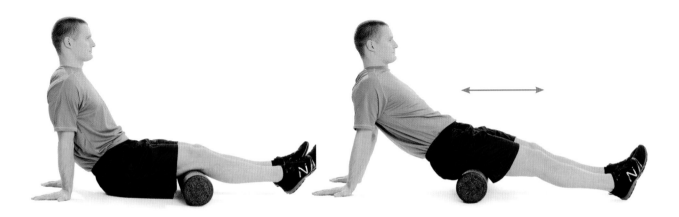

1 Sit with both legs straight out in front of you with the foam roller under your upper legs. Place your arms on the ground behind you to prop your upper body up off the floor.

2 Roll up and down the upper legs between the hips and knees. If you feel a spot that's tender or tight, spend more time working that particular area. Perform the roll for 15 to 30 seconds.

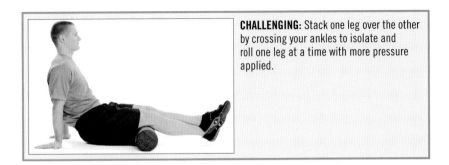

CHALLENGING: Stack one leg over the other by crossing your ankles to isolate and roll one leg at a time with more pressure applied.

Hamstring Front Leg Swing

Dynamic movements allow the use of controlled momentum to exaggerate our range of motion, thereby creating more elasticity in the muscle. This stretch warms up the hamstring muscle and is excellent for activities that require kicking or fast leg movements.

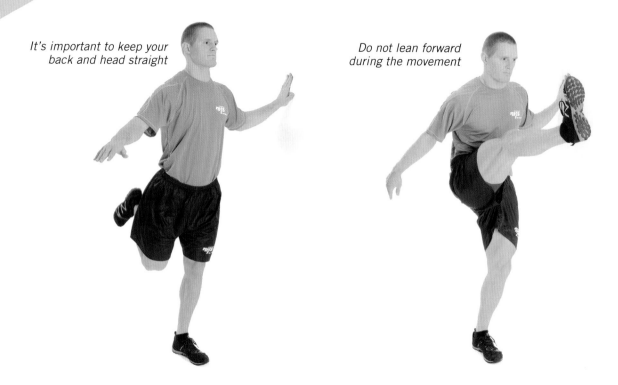

It's important to keep your back and head straight

Do not lean forward during the movement

1. Support your body with your left foot planted and left hand on a wall or doorway. In a continuous flow, bend your right leg behind you and kick it forward until it's fully extended. Bend the leg back to the start position. Start with a range of motion well within your comfort zone and gradually increase the speed and height of the kick. Repeat this movement for one set of 8 to 12 reps on each leg.

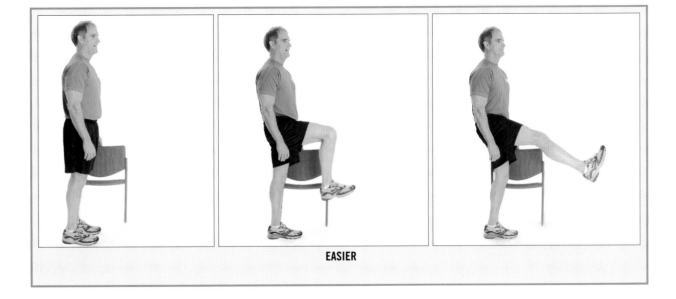

EASIER

TIP: This dynamic stretch is meant to warm up hamstrings just before an activity, and it should mimic the speed and range of motion that will be used in the activity.

Walking Hamstring Stretch

Dynamic movements are very important to complete prior to an activity. This stretch properly warms up the hamstrings for any activity that involves walking, running, bending, or sitting, to name only a few.

It's important to keep your back and head straight

Keep your knee as straight as possible

 1 Stand with your feet shoulder width apart and arms at your sides. Keep your core engaged and posture aligned throughout the movement.

2 Fully extend your right arm and left leg in front of your body. Keep your leg as straight as possible and your toe pointed toward the ceiling. The movement should be fairly slow and controlled.

3 Return your right arm to your side and your left leg to the floor as you move forward. Switch sides by extending your left arm and right leg in front of your body to complete the stretch on the opposite side. Continue the sequence for 8 to 10 reps on each leg.

CHALLENGING: For a deeper stretch once your muscles are warmed up, progressively speed up the movement with a faster, more continuous leg lift.

Lateral Lunge

Most of our lower body locomotive efforts occur in the forward direction during our daily activities. This leads to underuse of the inner and outer leg muscles, causing tightness and weakness in the upper leg. This stretch improves the mobility of these muscles that play an important role in hip strength and balance.

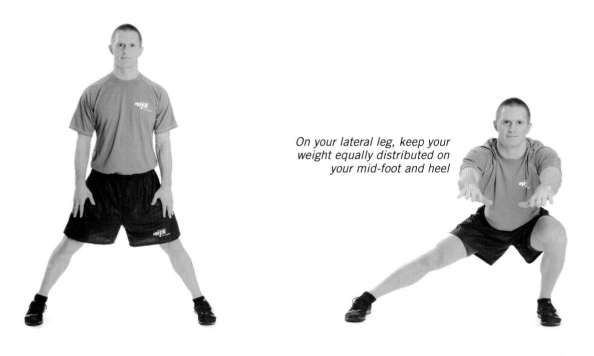

On your lateral leg, keep your weight equally distributed on your mid-foot and heel

1 Start by standing with your feet positioned flat on the floor, wider than shoulder width apart, and your arms relaxed at your sides.

2 Extend your arms in front of your body as you lift your left leg and take a lateral step 2 to 3 feet to the left. Keep your right leg straight as you press your hips back. Feel the stretch along your upper thighs. Return to the starting position. Repeat the lunge on the right side and complete 8 to 12 reps on each leg.

> **CAUTION:** Your knee should stay aligned with your ankle during the stretch.

Backward Lunge

The lunge is an incredibly beneficial lower body strengthening exercise. It also provides a great stretch for the upper leg. Combining the lunge with a backward step improves the flexibility of the hip, thigh, and calf muscles, and challenges your balance.

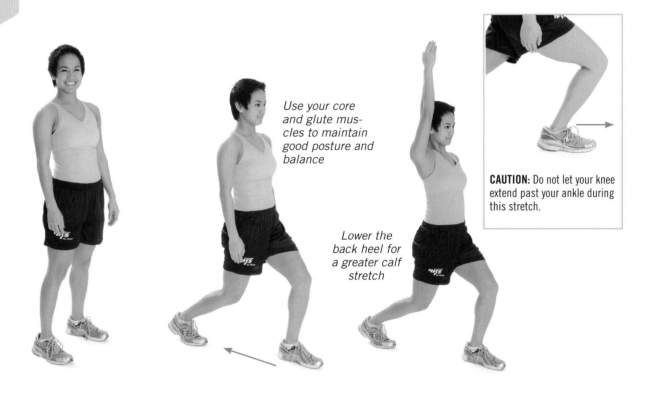

Use your core and glute muscles to maintain good posture and balance

Lower the back heel for a greater calf stretch

CAUTION: Do not let your knee extend past your ankle during this stretch.

1 Stand straight and tall with your weight evenly distributed on both feet. With your glute muscles squeezed tight, initiate the movement with your right glute to lift and pull the right leg behind you.

2 Use your left glute and thigh muscles to balance and move into the lowered position. Extend your right arm overhead as you distribute your body weight over both legs. Return to the start position by shifting your weight to the forward leg and pulling the back leg forward. Repeat this movement on the opposite leg and alternate for 6 to 10 repetitions on each leg.

Lying Side Quadriceps Stretch

Among the largest and most called-upon muscles in the body, the quadriceps tend to become tight, which can gradually lead to back and knee pain. This is a gentle stretch that can improve flexibility in the leg and hip and help alleviate pain.

 Lie on your left side with your left arm on the floor under your ear. Your right arm should be resting on the right side with your legs stacked one on the other.

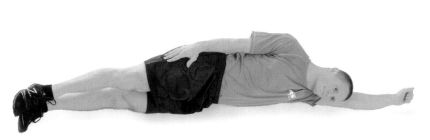

> **CAUTION:** Don't compensate for tight quads by arching your back to pull your leg behind you.

2 To complete the stretch, bring your right heel as close to your buttocks as possible. Place your right hand around your lower leg to hold the stretch. Your knees should remain close together. Repeat on the opposite side.

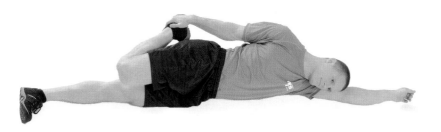

> **TIP:** If you're not able to reach your lower leg with your hand, use a towel or rope for assistance.

Standing Quadriceps Stretch

The quadriceps are four muscles along the front of your thigh. They work with the hamstrings to stabilize your knee and pelvis. The quads are responsible for extending the leg at the knee and raising the leg at the hip.

For support, stand near a wall or sturdy piece of exercise equipment

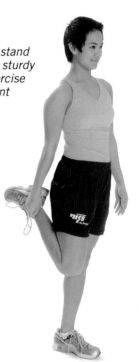
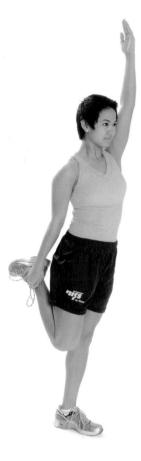

1 Holding your ankle, gently pull your right heel toward your buttocks. Stand straight and tall and tighten your stomach muscles to prevent your back from arching.

2 Gently pull up on your right leg until you feel tension in your thigh. Extend your left arm overhead as you move into the stretch. Keep your knees close together. Hold for 15 to 20 seconds and repeat on the opposite side.

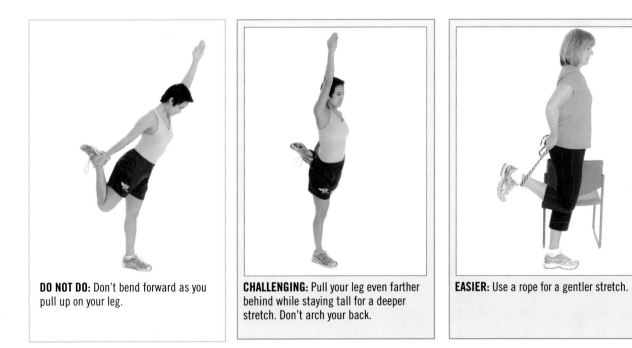

DO NOT DO: Don't bend forward as you pull up on your leg.

CHALLENGING: Pull your leg even farther behind while staying tall for a deeper stretch. Don't arch your back.

EASIER: Use a rope for a gentler stretch.

Standing Hamstring Stretch

Some of the most effective stretches for relieving low back pain work the hamstrings. This is because the hamstring muscles attach to the pelvis and run down the back of the thigh to the knee. Tight hamstrings restrict movement in the pelvis, put pressure on the surrounding structures, and can lead to debilitating injuries.

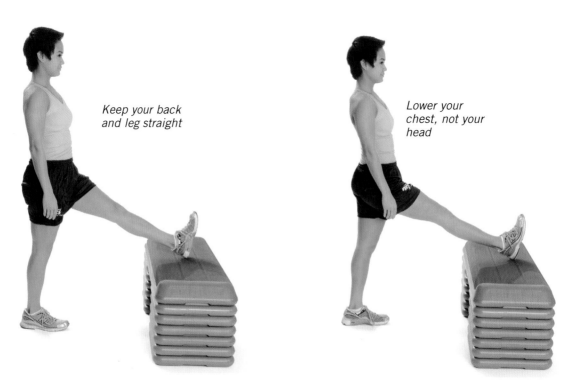

Keep your back and leg straight

Lower your chest, not your head

1 With your left leg extended and toes pointed upward, elevate your leg on a moderately high surface. Stand straight and tall and bend forward slightly until you feel a gentle stretch in the low back and hamstrings. Hold for 5 seconds, relax, and repeat, trying to increase the stretch each time. Accumulate 30 seconds of stretch and repeat on the opposite leg.

Seated One Leg Hamstring Stretch

Whether you bike, run, or are deskbound most of the day, it's important to give your hamstrings some TLC. As an extra bonus, this stretch will not only make your hamstrings happy, but your back, hips, and knees will thank you, too.

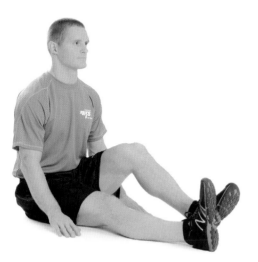

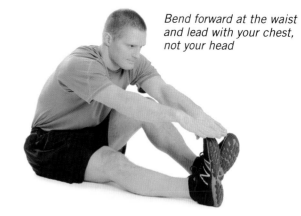

Bend forward at the waist and lead with your chest, not your head

1 Sit tall on the floor with your core tight and back straight, legs extended in front. Keep your right leg straight and your left leg slightly bent.

2 Feel the stretch throughout your right hamstring muscle by reaching toward your toes with both arms. Reach as far as you can without straining or lifting your left buttock off the floor. Hold for 15 to 20 seconds and repeat with the left leg extended.

CHALLENGING: Pull your heel closer to your buttocks and bend forward past the thigh.

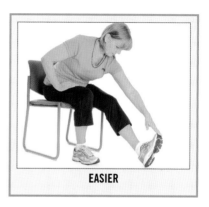

EASIER

Quadriceps Rope Stretch

The quads are the workhorses of the legs. As such, when they're not happy, you're not happy. While other quad exercises help you get limber before an activity, this stretch is most effective after exercise, when your muscles are warm. The rope not only offers a more complete range of motion, it's also a great tool for those with limited shoulder mobility.

 Lie flat on your stomach with the rope wrapped around your right foot and both ends in your right hand.

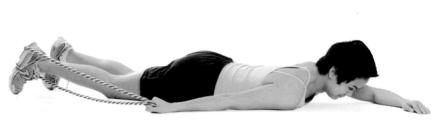

 Bring your right heel as close to your buttocks as possible by pulling the rope over your shoulder. Pull until you feel a gentle stretch in the upper thigh, and hold for 15 to 20 seconds. Repeat the stretch on the opposite leg.

Your knee should't leave the floor at any time during the stretch

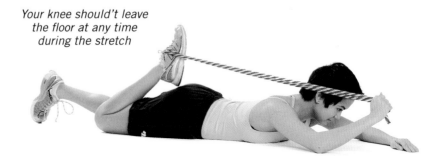

CHALLENGING: Hold the position of first resistance for 15 to 20 seconds. Then, without moving the leg, use the rope to contract the quadriceps for 3 to 5 seconds. Relax and immediately move into a greater range of motion. Repeat the contract/relax for 2 to 3 reps.

Hamstring Rope Stretch

This is a good stretch to increase the elasticity and range of motion in your hamstring muscles. Using the rope allows you to stretch the muscle through a greater range of motion. Over time this allows the hamstrings to move more freely. This is also an important stretch if you're experiencing low back pain.

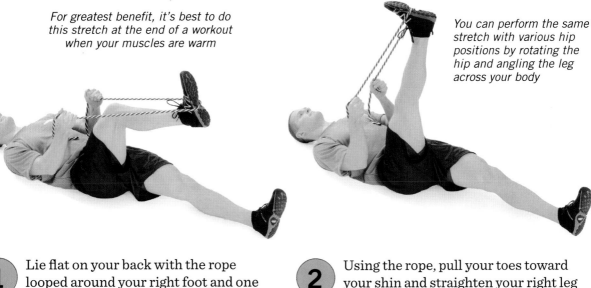

For greatest benefit, it's best to do this stretch at the end of a workout when your muscles are warm

You can perform the same stretch with various hip positions by rotating the hip and angling the leg across your body

1 Lie flat on your back with the rope looped around your right foot and one end in each hand. Start with your left leg extended on the floor and your right leg slightly bent.

2 Using the rope, pull your toes toward your shin and straighten your right leg toward the ceiling. Pull your leg to your torso as far as your hamstrings allow. Hold for 10 to 15 seconds and repeat 2 or 3 times, trying to pull a little farther each time. Repeat the stretch with the left leg.

CHALLENGING: Hold the position of first resistance for 15 to 20 seconds. Then, without moving the leg, use the rope to contract the hamstrings for 3 to 5 seconds. Relax and immediately move into a greater range of motion. Repeat the contract/relax 2 or 3 reps.

lower legs

Calf Foam Roll

The calf is one of the most used muscles in the body, bearing most of the body's weight when standing or moving. Tension and knots are common in this muscle and can be relieved using the foam roller.

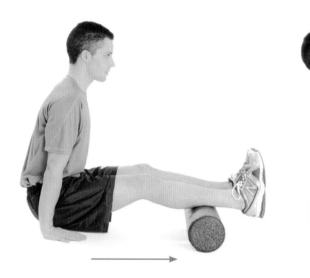

TIP: For a deeper massage, move one leg on top of the other and roll one calf at a time.

1 Sit on the ground with both legs out in front of you and place the roller under your lower legs. Use your arms as support to slightly raise your hips off the ground to keep your body perpendicular with the roller.

2 Roll back and forth over the lower leg muscles for 15 to 30 seconds. If a spot feels tender or sore, spend a little more time rolling that specific area.

Tibialis Anterior Foam Roll

A tight tibialis anterior is a contributing factor in shin splints. Tightness is often caused by overuse injuries from running or jumping. Using the foam roller to release some of the tension in the muscle can help alleviate symptoms of shin splints.

CAUTION: If you currently have shin splints, consult with a doctor before performing this movement.

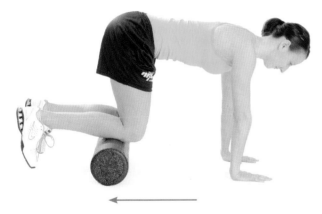

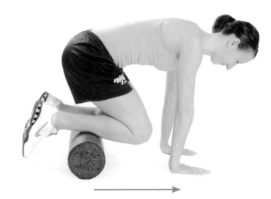

1 Place the foam roller just below the knees on the front of your lower leg. Keep your back in a flat table top position.

2 Using your hips to complete the movement, roll up and down the muscles on the outside of your shins between the knees and ankles. If you feel a spot that's extra tender or tight, focus on the spot and roll that area out a little longer. Continue this for 15 to 30 seconds.

Ankle Circles

Ankle sprains and strains are among the most common of all athletic injuries, yet can also happen when you simply step on an uneven surface. This dynamic stretch targets the many muscles, tendons, and ligaments responsible for your ease of movement, agility, and balance.

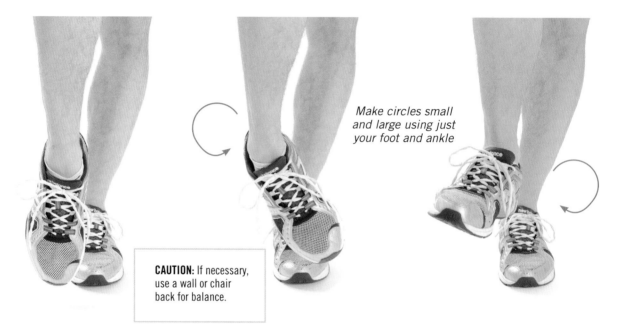

Make circles small and large using just your foot and ankle

CAUTION: If necessary, use a wall or chair back for balance.

1 Stand tall with your core engaged and glutes contracted. Lift one foot off the floor and make circles moving only the ankle joint. Circle slowly 8 to 10 times to the right and then 8 to 10 times to the left. Repeat on the other foot.

TIP: Engage your glute muscles to improve your balance on one foot.

Walking Toe Raise

Dynamic movements of the lower leg are important before an activity, as this part of the body bears most of the weight when standing and moving. This dynamic activity properly prepares the muscles of the lower leg for exercise.

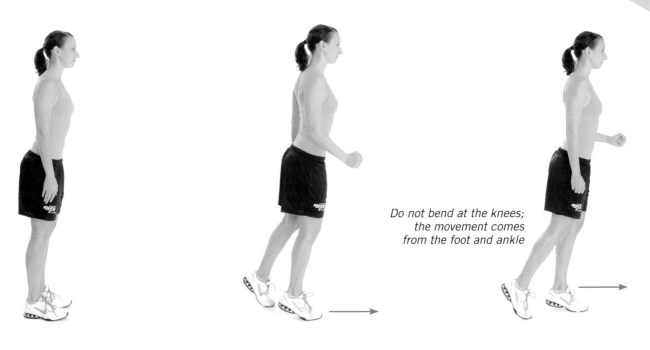

Do not bend at the knees; the movement comes from the foot and ankle

 1 Stand with your feet shoulder width apart and arms at your sides. Keep your core engaged and posture aligned throughout the movement.

2 With a slight bounce in your step, rise up onto your right toes and push off as you propel yourself forward. Rise up onto your left toes as you take the next step forward. Repeat from right to left for 8 to 12 repetitions on each leg

CHALLENGING: For a more strenuous stretch, slow your walking stride and circle your ankle as it reaches for the next step, while balancing on the toes of the opposite foot.

Standing Calf Stretch

Standing or pressing your foot on the gas pedal for long periods of time can lead to tightness in your lower leg muscles. This stretch can help alleviate some of this tightness and improve blood flow to the area.

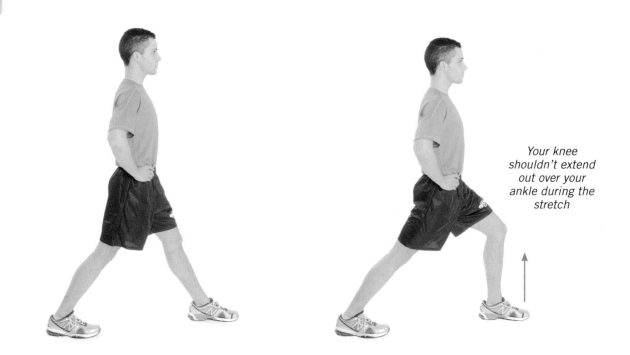

Your knee shouldn't extend out over your ankle during the stretch

1 Stand with your feet shoulder width apart with your left foot planted on the floor about 1 foot in front of you and your right foot about 1 foot behind you.

2 Maintaining good posture and keeping your feet flat on the floor, shift your weight as you bend your left leg forward. Allow the right leg to extend, feeling a gentle stretch in the lower leg. Hold for 15 to 20 seconds and repeat with the opposite leg.

Kneeling One Leg Calf Stretch

With the lower leg bearing much of the weight of the body, it's important to maintain flexibility in the calf muscles. Tightness in this area can lead to improper form in locomotive activities such as walking and running, which can result in injury. Use this stretch to improve flexibility in the lower leg.

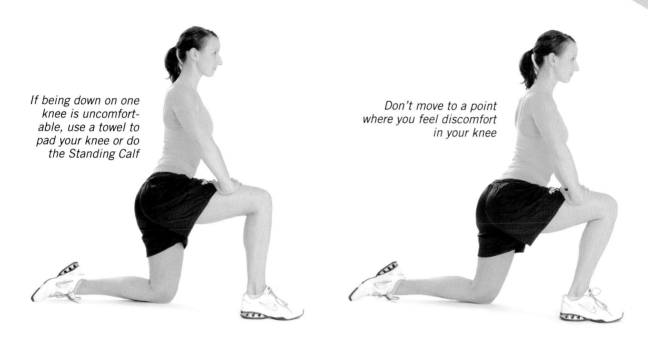

If being down on one knee is uncomfortable, use a towel to pad your knee or do the Standing Calf

Don't move to a point where you feel discomfort in your knee

 1 Kneel on your left knee with the left leg on the floor behind and your right leg bent in front of you. Your hands should be resting on your right leg, and your core should be tight with your posture properly aligned.

2 Move into the stretch by shifting your right knee forward while maintaining good posture. When you feel a gentle tension in the lower right leg, hold for 15 to 20 seconds. Repeat the stretch on the other side.

Gastrocnemius Rope Stretch

Shin splints are a common athletic injury that can lead to time off from sports in order to heal. Stretching the muscles of the lower leg can help prevent some cases of shin splints, and is also recommended in later stages of rehab from an injury. This assisted stretch is excellent for both purposes.

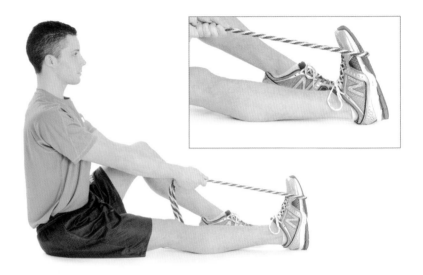

1 Sit on the floor with your left leg extended in front of you, toe pointed upward, and your right leg bent with the foot flat on the floor. Wrap the rope around the mid-foot of your right leg and hold one end in each hand. Keep your core tight and spine properly aligned.

2 Pull the rope, moving your toe toward the front of your lower leg. When you feel a deep stretch in the calf muscle, don't pull the rope any farther. Hold for 15 to 20 seconds and repeat on the other leg.

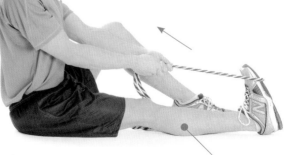

CAUTION: If you currently have shin splints, consult with a doctor before proceeding with the stretch.

Feel it here

Calf Rope Stretch

Assisted stretches help to improve flexibility by further challenging the normal range of motion of a muscle. Using the rope to stretch the calf gives a deeper stretch than you can achieve on your own.

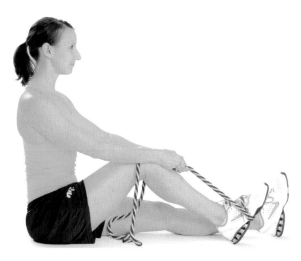 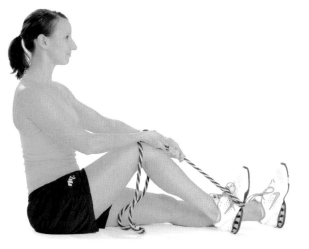

1 Sit on the floor with both legs extended out in front, with your core tight and spine properly aligned. Wrap the rope around the mid-foot of your right leg and bend the leg up slightly. Hold one end of the rope in each hand between your knee and ankle.

2 Pull the rope, moving your toe to point toward the ceiling. When you feel a deep stretch in the calf muscle, don't pull the rope any further. Hold this stretch for 15 to 20 seconds and repeat on the other leg.

whole
body

Standing One Leg Rotation

If you're looking for an advanced challenge for balance and flexibility, this is the stretch for you! This incorporates strength, single leg balance, and a stretch through your sides to make it beneficial to many muscle groups.

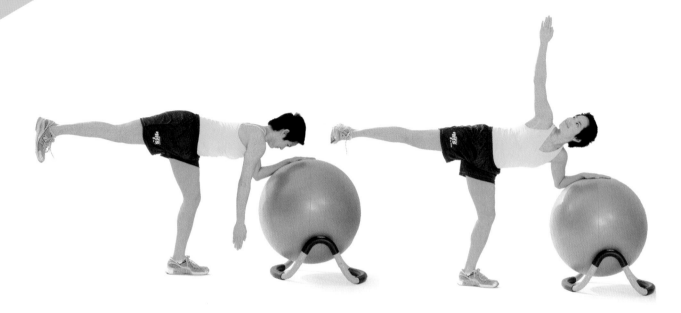

1 Using a supported stability ball, place your left hand on the ball with your right arm extended to the floor. Keeping your left leg planted with a slight bend at your knee, extend your right leg behind. Keep your core tight for the duration of the stretch.

2 Complete the pose by turning your torso and reaching your right arm up toward the ceiling. Turn as far as is comfortable while maintaining balance until you feel the stretch. Hold this pose for 10 to 15 seconds and repeat on the opposite side.

CAUTION: This is an advanced stretch and should be performed only by those who feel they have adequate balance.

Opposite One Arm One Leg Reach

Maintaining stability and balance becomes more challenging as we age. Performing movements that promote stability is important for long-term fitness and independence. This whole body stretch provides the benefit of flexibility throughout the body.

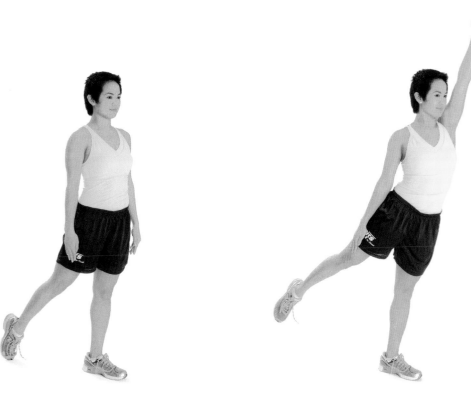

 1 Maintain good posture with your core tight and arms relaxed at your sides. Start with your left foot planted on the floor and your right foot behind your body resting on the toes.

 2 Keeping your torso squared, raise your left arm overhead and extend your right leg behind by raising the foot off the floor. Reach upward as far as you can with your arm and behind with your leg while maintaining good balance. Hold for 10 to 15 seconds and repeat on the opposite side.

EASIER: For those with poor balance, start by keeping both feet on the floor.

One Leg Balanced Reach and Rotation

Lateral movement and balance are important for sports such as skiing, soccer, and basketball. They're also needed for daily activities such as sweeping. This movement challenges the body to move laterally in multiple directions while staying balanced.

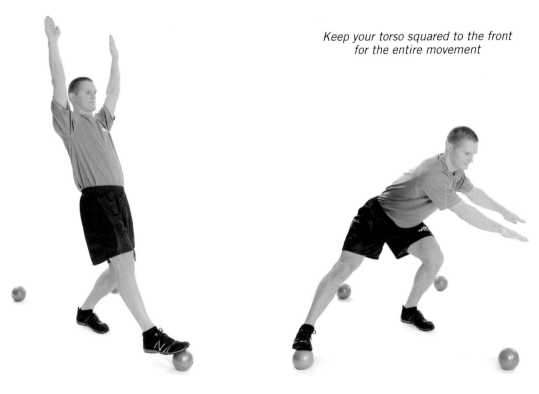

Keep your torso squared to the front for the entire movement

1 Position four objects equidistant around you 2 to 3 feet from the center, placing one straight in front, one straight behind, one to the left, and one to the right to set up this movement. Stand in the middle of the four objects. Balanced on your left leg for the entire movement, start by reaching your right foot to the front object as you extend your arms overhead.

2 Return to the start position and reach your right foot to the right object as you extend your arms to the left.

CHALLENGING: When you're comfortable with the movement and are looking for a more challenging stretch, move the objects a little farther from the center to extend your reach.

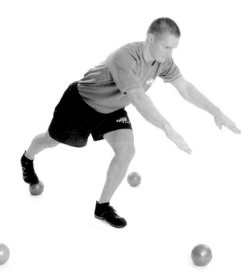 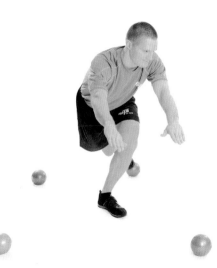

3 Return to the start position and reach your right foot to the object behind as you extend your arms to the front.

4 Return to the start position and reach your right foot to the left object as you extend your arms to the right. Repeat this sequence 4 to 8 times and then switch sides by balancing on the right leg and reaching with the left foot.

Over and Under Medicine Ball Squat

Humans have been picking things up and carrying them overhead for thousands of years. In today's world we're not required to do that as much as we would have years ago. This exercise will help improve flexibility and strength needed to lift objects high.

Press your hips back to get into the squat position

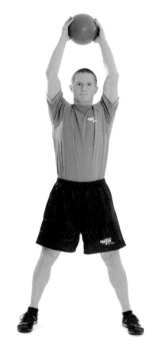

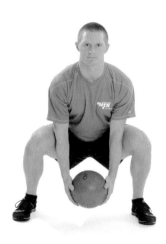

EASIER

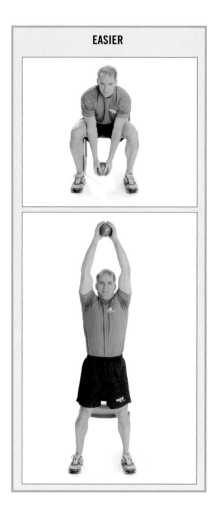

 1 Begin in a squat position with your feet wider than shoulder width apart, arms extended between your legs, holding a medicine ball with both hands. Your core should be tight and back straight throughout the movement.

2 As you stand up from the squat position, extend your arms overhead. Reach the ball as high as is comfortable and pause before returning to the start position. Repeat this movement 8 to 12 times.

CAUTION: Your knees should not cross over your toes during the squat phase of the movement.

Warrior 1 Pose

Not only is this a great full body stretch, it strengthens, improves balance, reinforces correct posture, and rejuvenates the entire body as well. Notice the benefits especially in the legs, torso, and shoulders.

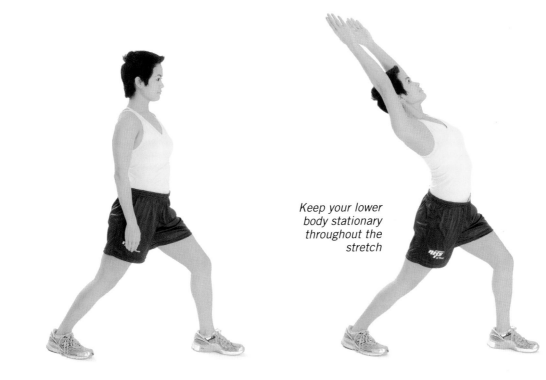

Keep your lower body stationary throughout the stretch

1 With your core tight and arms relaxed at your sides, begin with your feet shoulder width apart and then stagger them so your left foot is in front and right foot behind 3 to 4 feet apart. Your left leg should be slightly bent and the right almost fully extended.

2 Keeping your torso squared forward, fully extend both arms overhead as you arch your torso back, pressing your chest out in front. Feel the stretch through your whole body, and hold for 15 to 20 seconds.

CAUTION: Do not extend past the point of comfort for this pose. If you feel any pain with this stretch, do not continue.

Warrior 2 Pose

A great stretch for the sides of the body, Warrior 2 provides improved balance, strength, and flexibility through the inner and outer thighs, obliques, and shoulders.

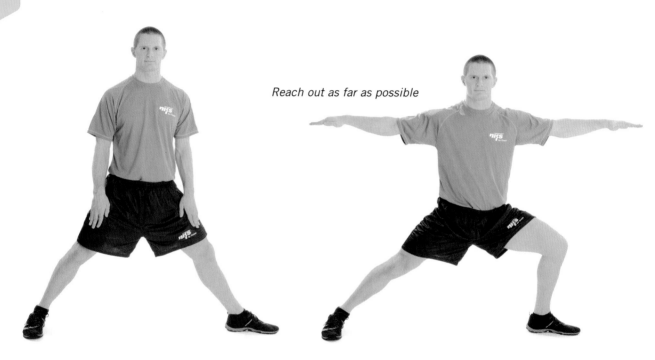

Reach out as far as possible

1 With your core tight and arms relaxed at your sides, begin with your feet wider than shoulder width apart with your right foot pointed forward and your left foot pointed out to the side. Your upper body should remain squared forward throughout the movement.

2 Raise both arms out to the sides extended fully. Lunge laterally to the left by extending your right leg and bending your left knee until you feel the stretch throughout the body. Hold this pose for 15 to 20 seconds and repeat on the opposite side.

Golfer's Rotation with Ball

An essential component of the golf swing is adequate rotation of the shoulders, hips, and back. Without this ability it's difficult to get into the proper position for the start and follow-through of the swing. This movement helps to improve the flexibility needed for an efficient swing.

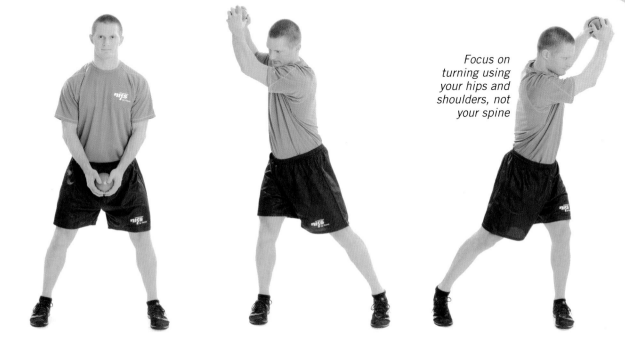

Focus on turning using your hips and shoulders, not your spine

1 Start in good posture with your feet wider than shoulder width apart, holding a small ball with both hands. Hold the ball in the middle of the body with your arms relaxed at the front.

2 Rotate to the right turning your left shoulder over your right. Lift your left heel off the floor as a pivot to rotate. Rotate back as far as is comfortable and hold for a few seconds before returning to the start position.

3 Next rotate to the left turning your right shoulder over your left, using your right foot as a pivot to assist. Rotate as far as is comfortable and hold for a few seconds before returning to the start position. Repeat this sequence 8 to 12 times.

Bent Knee Side Angle Pose

With many of our daily movements and activities performed in the frontal plane of the body, flexibility and strength in the sides isn't first on our mind. This stretch does both, as well as utilize balance skills for the sides of the body ranging from the shoulders down to the legs.

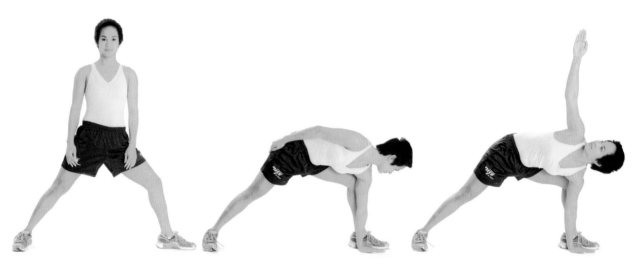

1 Stand tall with straight posture, arms relaxed at your sides, and feet wider than shoulder width apart. Turn your left leg out by moving your left foot out away from the left side of your body.

2 Keeping both feet on the floor, reach your left hand down toward the floor as you bend your left leg lower to the ground.

3 Turn your torso and head toward the ceiling, reaching up with your right arm. Keep your left hand flat on the floor for the duration of the stretch. Hold this pose for 10 to 15 seconds.

EASIER: If you have limited flexibility, use a prop such as a box or block to elevate your hand higher off the floor to perform the stretch.

Downward Facing Dog

A common yoga pose, Downward Facing Dog provides a plethora of benefits for the entire body, from the wrists to the ankles. It's an easy relaxation pose and also benefits strength and posture throughout the entire body.

Keep your back flat throughout the stretch

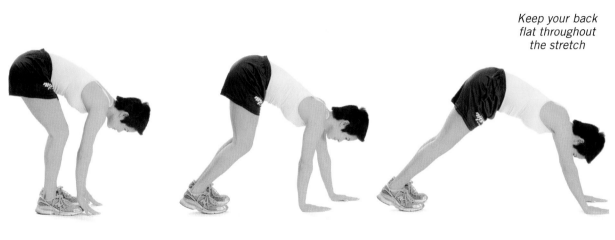

1 Start this pose with your feet shoulder width apart, your knees slightly bent, and your fingers on the floor.

2 Walk your hands in front of you, keeping your back flat as you lengthen your legs and rise up onto your toes.

3 Hold the stretch for 10 to 15 seconds after you've reached the final position with your legs and arms extended as far as is comfortable and hips up toward the ceiling.

CAUTION: Do not extend past the point of comfort for this pose or round out your back to fully extend the legs.

Inch Worm

The Inch Worm is an excellent dynamic warm-up for the entire back side of the body, especially the hamstrings, back, calves, and shoulders. Do this before any type of physical activity to see improved mobility.

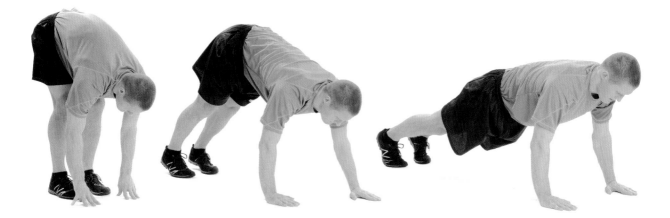

1 Begin with your feet shoulder width apart and bend the knees so your fingers are on the floor. Slowly walk your hands out in front of your body into a plank position, lengthening your back and hamstrings.

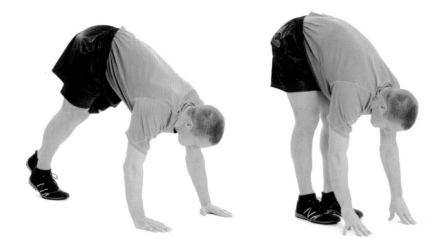

2 From the plank position, walk your feet up toward your hands, keeping your legs as straight as possible. When you start to feel your knees bend excessively, walk your hands forward again. Repeat the sequence 8 to 10 times.

Part 3

Stretching Routines

In this part, you'll find a variety of stretching routines geared toward specific activities and sports. The individual stretches listed in each routine can be found in Part 2. It's best to try completing the whole routine in the order it's listed, but if you have limited time you can pick and choose from the routine.

As stated in Part 1, the amount of time to hold the stretch and how many times you repeat the stretch will vary based on your fitness level and available time.

The majority of these routines should take between 10 to 25 minutes to complete. If you don't find a routine that suits your needs, use this section as a guide to develop your own or pick an activity routine that incorporates similar movements and muscles.

Keep your flexibility program interesting and challenging by frequently trying new routines or swapping out a few stretches here and there. Your muscles will respond better when hit with stretches from different angles, and your mind will appreciate a fresh routine now and then.

Regardless how you mix your stretches, remember to always stretch muscles when they're warm, follow dynamic movements with static stretches, and include foam roller exercises at the beginning or end of the routine.

Active Warm-Up Movements

This is how it all begins. Replace any type of "old style" stretching you did as a warm-up with these dynamic movements. Start these after 5 to 10 minutes of gentle cardiovascular exercise such as fast walking, light jogging, or rowing. It's commonly believed that active or dynamic stretches can aid in injury prevention when performed prior to an activity. This is an excellent dynamic routine to work all the major muscle groups to prepare for most sports.

Time: Beginner: 5–15 minutes
Intermediate: 10–20 minutes
Advanced: 15–25 minutes

Areas targeted: Wrists, Shoulders, Chest, Lower Leg, Ankles, Upper Leg, Hips, Lower Back

Props: Stability Ball

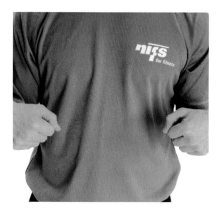

Wrist Circles

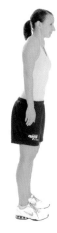

Shoulder Roll

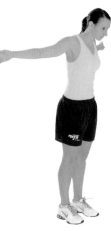

Dynamic Chest Movement

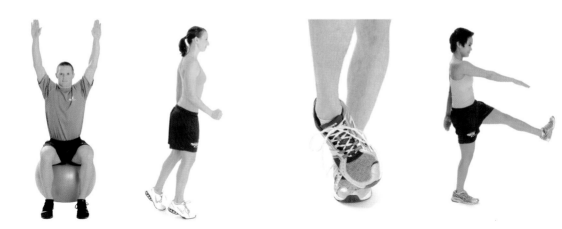

Dynamic Overhead Reach   Walking Toe Raise   Ankle Circles   Walking Hamstring Stretch

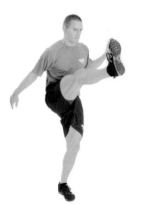

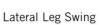

Hamstring Front Leg
Swing   Lateral Leg Swing   Forward Lunge Forearm to
Instep   Spinal Rotation

Tight Beginner

Many people are drawn to stretching because they feel tight; if this is true for you, don't be intimidated by the stretches in this book. Look for the modifications highlighted on many stretches, and remember that in the beginning, a partial stretch is better than no stretch at all. For those new to stretching, this routine combines multiple beginner poses in a series of gentle stretches, and is a great program to get you started with a full body stretch.

Time: Beginner: 5–15 minutes
Intermediate: 10–25 minutes
Advanced: 15–40 minutes

Areas targeted: Shoulders, Arms, Chest, Core, Hips, Lower Leg, Upper Leg, Lower Back

Props: None

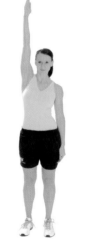

Overhead Shoulder Reach

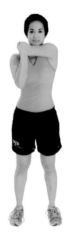

Bent Arm Triceps Crossover

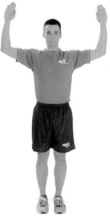

Bent Arm Fly

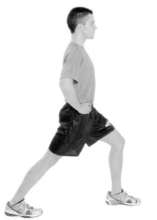

Standing Calf Stretch

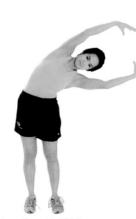

Standing Half Moon

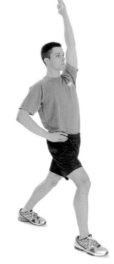

Standing Hip Flexor Stretch

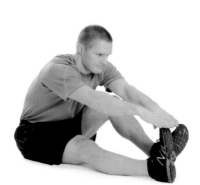

Seated Hamstring Stretch with Leg
Extended

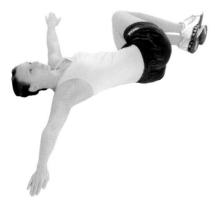

Spinal Rotation

The Morning Stretch

This quick 5- to 10-minute routine before you even get out of bed will set the tone for a productive day. Generally, the muscles of the back, shoulders, and neck are tightest when you first wake up. These stretches will awaken your senses and get your blood flowing and your mind alert. Who wouldn't like to start their day that way? Take your time and focus on your movements and breathing.

Time: Beginner: 5–15 minutes
Intermediate: 10–25 minutes
Advanced: 15–40 minutes

Areas targeted: Lower Back, Upper Back, Lower Leg, Neck, Shoulders, Ankles

Props: Stability Ball

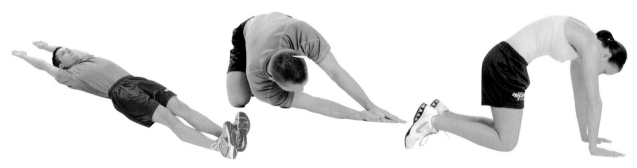

Lying Full Body Reach   Extended Arm Child's Pose   Cat and Camel

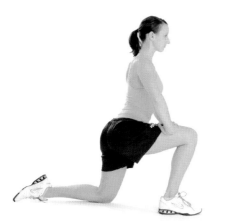

Kneeling One Leg Calf Stretch

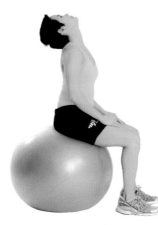

Neck Extension

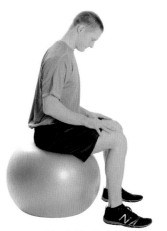

Neck Flexion

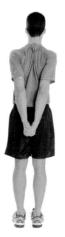

Behind Back Shoulder Reach

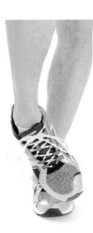

Ankle Circles

The Evening Stretch

The goal of this routine is to quietly unwind, relax the mind, and release the day's tension. These simple moves will help you find relaxation, balance, and flexibility at the end of a long day. Make the evening stretch your prelude to a good night's sleep, along with your favorite warm drink and some soothing music.

Time: Beginner: 5–15 minutes
Intermediate: 10–25 minutes
Advanced: 15–40 minutes

Areas targeted: Neck, Shoulders, Hips, Upper Back, Lower Back

Props: Risers

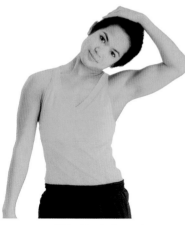

Side Neck Stretch

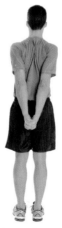

Behind Back Shoulder Reach

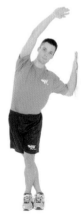

Standing Outer Hip Stretch

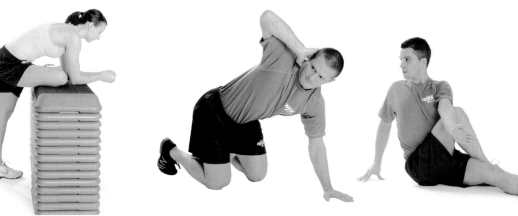

Standing Piriformis Stretch   Kneeling Rotation   Seated Leg Crossover

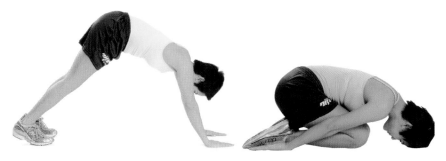

Downward Facing Dog   Child's Pose

The Quick 6

These six stretches can be squeezed into even the most chaotic of schedules. This routine not only can be completed in just a few minutes, it can be done virtually anywhere with a bit of open space. Focusing on many of the major muscle groups, you will notice benefits throughout the body. While you will want a more in-depth stretching routine most days of the week, the Quick Six is a perfect workout for those days when your time is limited.

Time: Beginner: 5–10 minutes
Intermediate: 5–15 minutes
Advanced: 10–20 minutes

Areas targeted: Arms, Chest, Lower Back, Core, Upper Leg, Hips

Props: None

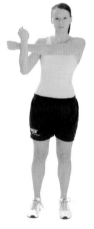

Straight Arm Crossover

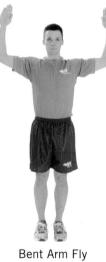

Bent Arm Fly

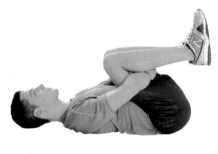

Double Knees to Chest

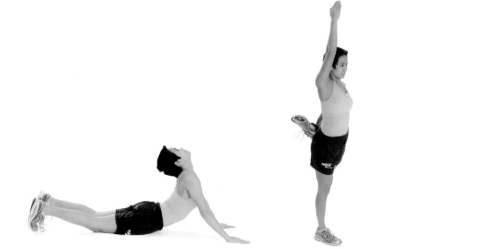

Lying Chest Lift (Cobra)   Standing Quad Stretch   Standing Hip Flexor Stretch

The Daily Dozen

Are you an overachiever by nature? Here are 12 stretches that will improve your range of motion from head to toe. Dedicate 30 to 60 minutes to this routine to gain the most benefit. While it may at first take a bit longer than most other routines, you'll soon notice how smoothly you can move from one stretch to another in this full-body workout.

Time: Beginner: 10–20 minutes
Intermediate: 10–30 minutes
Advanced: 20–60 minutes

Areas targeted: Neck, Shoulders, Arms, Chest, Upper Back, Lower Back, Core, Upper Leg, Lower Leg

Props: Rope, Risers

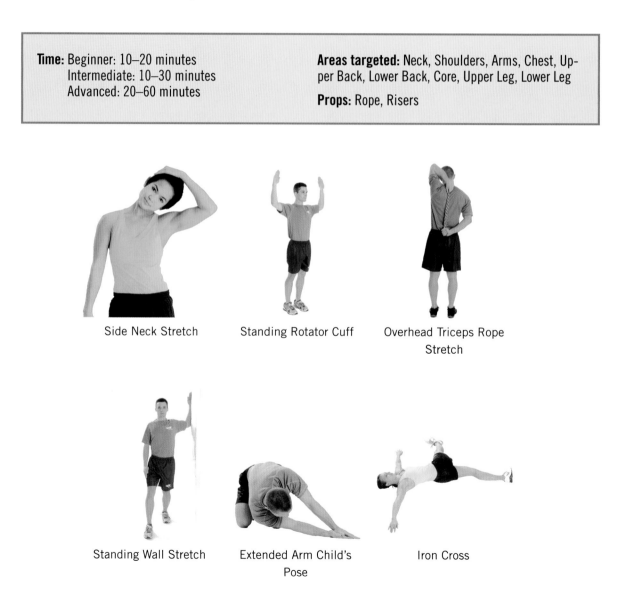

Side Neck Stretch

Standing Rotator Cuff

Overhead Triceps Rope Stretch

Standing Wall Stretch

Extended Arm Child's Pose

Iron Cross

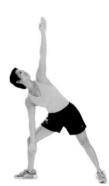

Triangle Pose

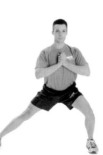

Lateral Lunge

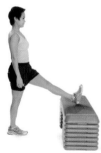

Standing One Leg
Hamstring Stretch

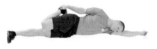

Lying Side Quadriceps
Stretch

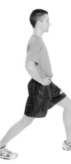

Standing Calf Stretch

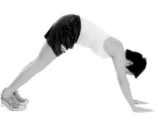

Downward Facing Dog

Stretching for Relaxation

Stretching can be a powerful tool in the management of physical and emotional stress. Once you know how your relaxed muscles feel, it becomes much easier to release built-up tension with a few targeted stretches. These stretches deliver overall body relaxation and put you on the track toward more progressive stress-relieving exercise.

Time: Beginner: 5–15 minutes
Intermediate: 10–25 minutes
Advanced: 15–40 minutes

Areas targeted: Neck, Shoulders, Upper Back, Lower Back, Core, Hips

Props: None

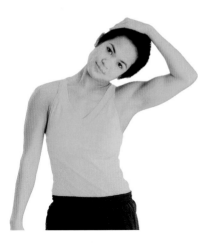

Side Neck Stretch

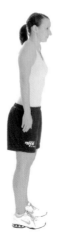

Shoulder Roll

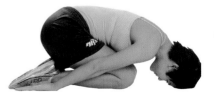

Child's Pose

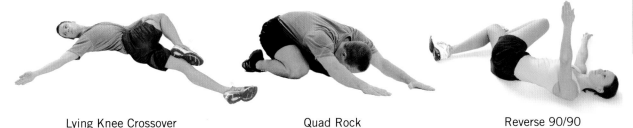

Lying Knee Crossover   Quad Rock   Reverse 90/90

Downward Dog   Lying Chest Lift (Cobra)

Stretching for Better Posture

Proper posture is more than just sitting and standing straight. It involves opening your chest and lengthening your spine, both of which help you breathe easier and reduce strain on your back. Keep in mind that this 15-minute routine cannot offset 8 hours a day of being slouched in a chair. Focus on good posture all day long and target the muscles that need the most work with this routine.

Time: Beginner: 5–15 minutes
Intermediate: 10–25 minutes
Advanced: 15–40 minutes

Areas targeted: Shoulders, Upper Back, Lower Back, Whole Body

Props: Stability Ball

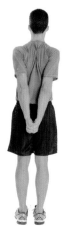

Behind Back Shoulder Reach

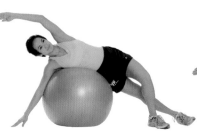

Lying Side Reach on Stability Ball

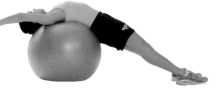

Back Extension on Stability Ball

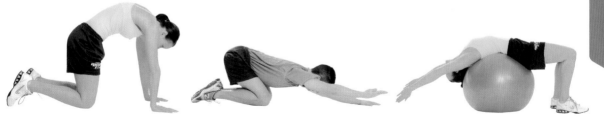

Cat and Camel   Kneeling Reach, Roll, and Lift   Stability Ball Back Release

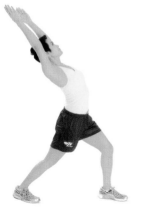

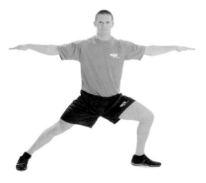

Warrior 1   Warrior 2

Stretching for Better Posture

Gardening

Gardening is great exercise, but just as you prepare for a workout, you need to prepare for the heavy lifting and endless bending and squatting. Before you reach for your tools, take a few minutes to warm up your muscles. As you're working, be sure to engage your core by actively drawing in your abdominal muscles when bending forward or twisting. Be aware of the signals your body is sending, and take short breaks to do some stretches.

Time: Beginner: 5–15 minutes
Intermediate: 10–25 minutes
Advanced: 15–40 minutes

Areas targeted: Neck, Wrists, Arms, Chest, Lower Back, Core, Hips

Props: Stability Ball

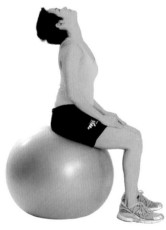

Neck Extension

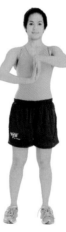

Wrist Flexion

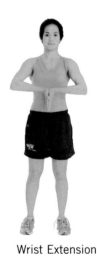

Wrist Extension

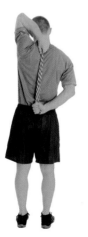

Overhead Triceps Rope Stretch

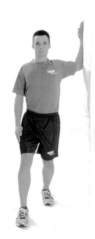

Standing Wall Stretch

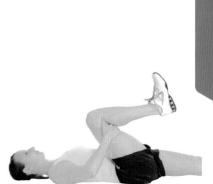

Single Knee to Chest

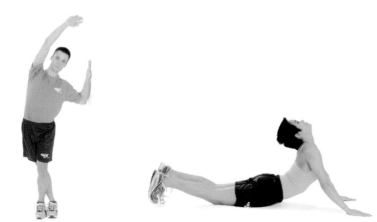

Standing Outer Hip Stretch

Lying Chest Lift (Cobra)

Deskercise at Work

The human body is not made to sit for long periods of time. Sitting at a desk, perhaps hunched over, typing and talking on the phone can lead to serious physical problems. The key is to stay mobile enough to prevent pain and stiffness. This routine does double duty by giving you a quick boost of energy and alertness. Remind yourself to take every opportunity to stand, walk, bend, twist, and just move at your desk.

Time: Beginner: 5–15 minutes
Intermediate: 10–25 minutes
Advanced: 15–40 minutes

Areas targeted: Wrists, Hands, Shoulders, Arms, Lower Back, Upper Leg

Props: Stability Ball

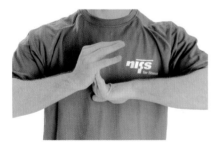

Finger Flexion/Extension

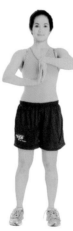

Wrist Flexion

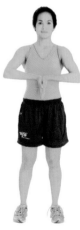

Wrist Extension

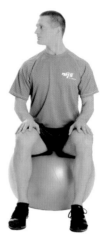

Side Neck Rotation

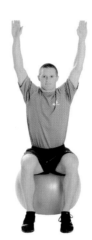

Dynamic Overhead Reach

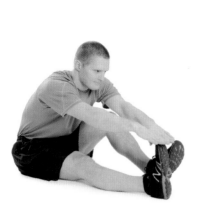

Seated Hamstring Stretch with Leg Extended

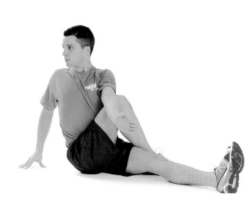

Seated Leg Crossover

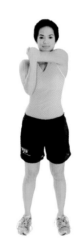

Bent Arm Triceps Crossover

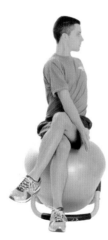

Seated Low Back Rotation

Standing for Long Periods

Standing in one place for a long time, even with good posture, can cause tightness and pain in muscles. The 24 moveable vertebrae that make up your spine are connected by ligaments and cushioned by intervertebral discs that function as shock absorbers and change shape as you move. Moving keeps your back healthy by pumping nutrients into the space. When standing for more than 15 minutes, remember that even small movements will help in minimizing back pain.

Time: Beginner: 5–15 minutes
Intermediate: 10–25 minutes
Advanced: 15–40 minutes

Areas targeted: Neck, Shoulders, Arms, Lower Back, Hips, Lower Legs

Props: Risers

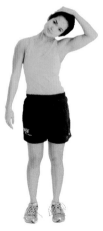

Side Neck Stretch

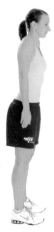

Shoulder Roll

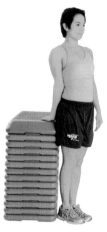

Front Arm Biceps Stretch

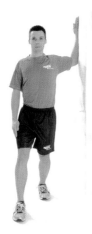

Standing Wall Stretch

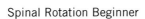

Spinal Rotation Beginner

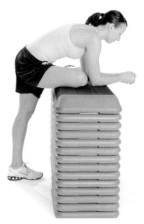

Standing Piriformis Stretch

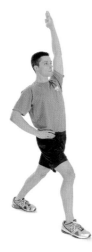

Standing Hip Flexor Stretch

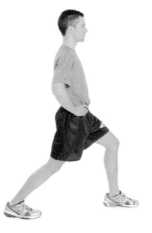

Standing Calf Stretch

Standing for Long Periods

Driving

Nothing can zap your flexibility and energy and leave your muscles stiff like a long drive. Combining better posture while driving with this series of gentle stretches before your trip and during stops can help you arrive at your destination feeling calm and relaxed. And don't underestimate the positive effect conscious deep breathing can have on your energy, stress level, and mental clarity during your drive.

Time: Beginner: 5–15 minutes
Intermediate: 10–25 minutes
Advanced: 15–40 minutes

Areas targeted: Wrists, Neck, Shoulders, Lower Back, Upper Leg, Lower Leg, Ankles

Props: Stability Ball

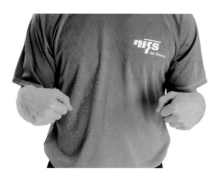

Wrist Circles

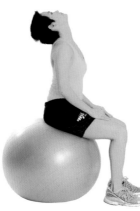

Neck Extension

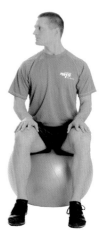

Side Neck Rotation

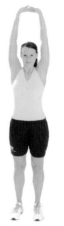

Overhead Shoulder Reach

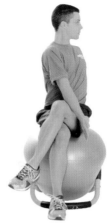

Seated Low Back Rotation

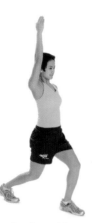

Backward Lunge

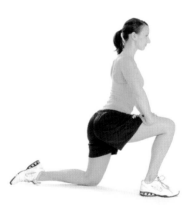

Kneeling One Leg Calf Stretch

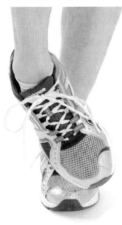

Ankle Circles

Stretching While Seated

There are plenty of good reasons to indulge in a seated stretching routine. This routine offers a great variety of stretches, and there's no need to get down on the floor! If you're unable to get up and move when you want, this series will help your stiffness and restlessness. If you're not comfortable with the stability ball, begin with a sturdy chair without wheels. Make sure your feet can firmly rest on the floor.

Time: Beginner: 5–15 minutes
Intermediate: 10–25 minutes
Advanced: 15–40 minutes

Areas targeted: Neck, Wrists, Arms, Upper Back, Lower Back, Hips, Upper Legs, Ankles

Props: Stability Ball

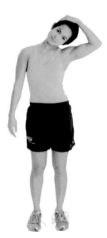

Side Neck Stretch

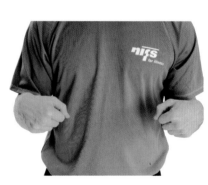

Wrist Circles

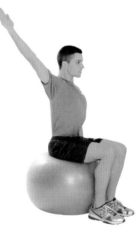

Seated Single Arm Chest Stretch

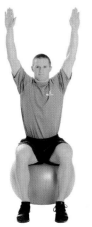

Dynamic Overhead Reach

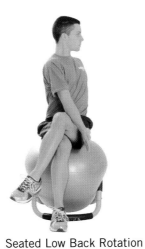

Seated Low Back Rotation

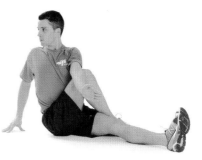

Seated Leg Crossover

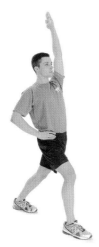

Standing Hip Flexor Stretch

Seated Hamstring Stretch with Leg
Extended

Foam Roller

A foam roller is an important tool for recovery. Your body adapts to the rigors of conditioning between workouts, so the more completely you recover, the better you'll feel in your next workout. Use a foam roller on any area that feels tight and in need of a massage. Roll the length of the muscle for as long as you feel it's productive. Foam rolling can be beneficial before or after a workout, or even while watching television.

Time: Beginner: 5–15 minutes
Intermediate: 10–25 minutes
Advanced: 15–40 minutes

Areas targeted: Chest, Upper Back, Lower Back, Upper Legs, Hips, Lower Legs

Props: Foam Roller

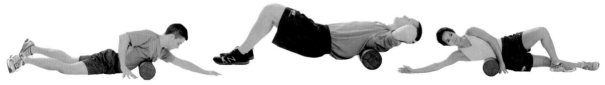

Chest Foam Roll   Upper Back Foam Roll   Lats Foam Roll

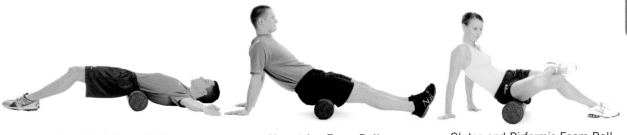

Low Back Foam Roll Hamstring Foam Roll Glutes and Pirformis Foam Roll

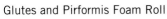

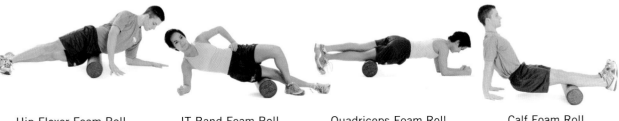

Hip Flexor Foam Roll IT Band Foam Roll Quadriceps Foam Roll Calf Foam Roll

Rope Stretches

Rope stretches are another important tool for muscle recovery. The rope can easily be found at a local hardware or home store. A 7- to 8-foot length works fine. The toughest part for most people is making the time for rope stretches, and stretching in general. Plan to make this a part of your exercise routine, and remember that this is done *after* a workout, when your muscles are warm.

Time: Beginner: 5–15 minutes
Intermediate: 10–25 minutes
Advanced: 15–40 minutes

Areas targeted: Arms, Hips, Upper Legs, Lower Legs

Props: Rope

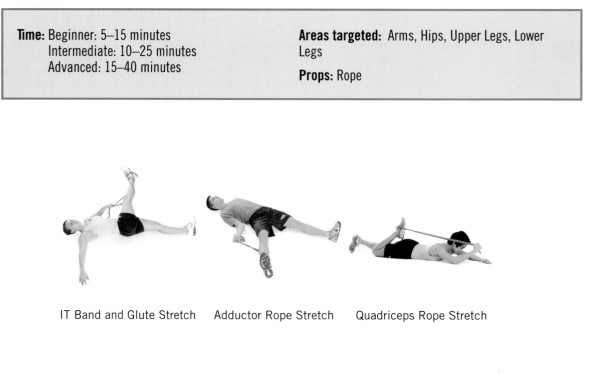

IT Band and Glute Stretch   Adductor Rope Stretch   Quadriceps Rope Stretch

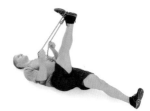   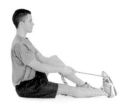   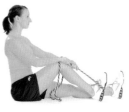   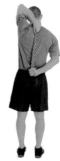

Hamstring Rope Stretch   Gastrocnemius Rope Stretch   Calf Rope Stretch   Overhead Triceps Rope Stretch

A Note on AIS

AIS is based on the scientific principle of reciprocal inhibition, which states that the muscle on one side of a joint must relax in order for the opposing muscle to contract. The technique has four basic steps:

1. *Isolate* the muscle to be stretched by actively contracting the opposite muscle. For instance, if you're stretching the hamstring you'll first contract the quadriceps. In doing this, the quadriceps will actually pull your leg up. When you feel your hamstring reach the end of its normal movement, apply gentle assistance with the rope and continue that range of motion by no more than 6 to 10 degrees.

2. *Hold* each stretch for no more than $1\frac{1}{2}$ to 2 seconds. This is critical in order to prevent activation of the stretch reflex (see "Beware of the Stretch Reflex" in Part 1).

3. *Repeat* each stretch 8 to 10 times for 1 or 2 sets. Always return the muscle being stretched to the starting position between reps. The repetitions are important in order to increase blood flow to the muscle being stretched.

4. *Exhale* during the stretch phase and inhale on the return phase.

Walking

Fitness walking can help you maintain a healthy weight; prevent or manage conditions such as Type 2 diabetes, heart disease, and high blood pressure; strengthen your bones; and improve your balance. Turn your casual walk into a fitness stride with good posture and a little intent. Focus on keeping your head up; relaxing your neck and shoulders; pumping your arms; tightening your stomach muscles; keeping your back tall; and rolling from heel to toe.

Time: Beginner: 5–15 minutes
Intermediate: 10–25 minutes
Advanced: 15–40 minutes

Areas targeted: Ankles, Upper Leg, Lower Leg, Hips, Lower Back, Shoulders

Props: None

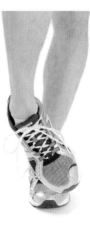

Ankle Circles

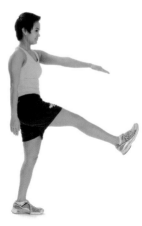

Walking Hamstring Stretch

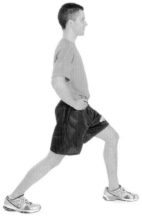

Standing Calf Stretch

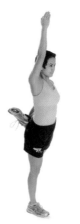

Standing Quadriceps Stretch

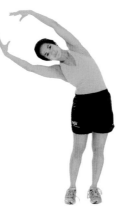

Standing Half Moon

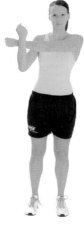

Straight Arm Crossover

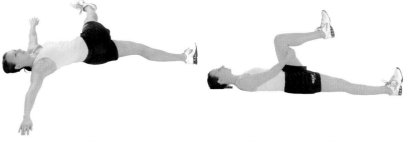

Iron Cross

Single Knee to Chest

Running

Runners often suffer from chronic tightness, in predictable areas—hamstrings, calf muscles, IT band, and quadriceps. While no stretching routine can offset the terrible toos—too much, too soon, too fast—the following stretches can give your joints greater flexibility in injury-prone areas. Remember to focus on the dynamic movements as part of your pre-activity warm-up, and the static and rope stretches after your workout when your muscles are warm.

Time: Beginner: 5–15 minutes
Intermediate: 10–25 minutes
Advanced: 15–40 minutes

Areas targeted: Upper Leg, Hips, Lower Leg, Lower Back, Core

Props: Risers

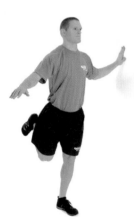

Hamstring Front Leg Swing

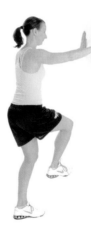

Lateral Leg Swing

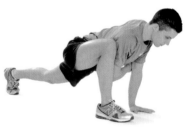

Forward Lunge Forearm to Instep

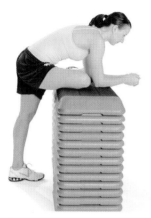

Standing Piriformis

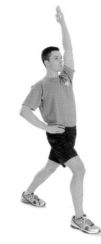

Standing Hip Flexor Stretch

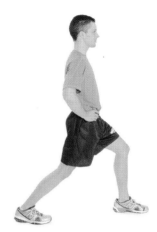

Standing Calf Stretch

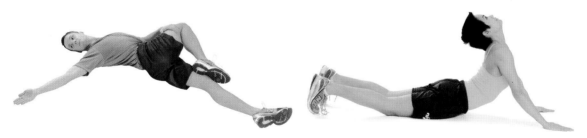

Lying Knee Crossover

Lying Chest Lift (Cobra)

Rowing

Rowing requires that you maintain a strong posture while generating a lot of power from the lower body. Your core muscles are crucial for this transfer of power from the legs to the oar. This is what makes rowing such a great whole-body exercise. It's also what makes it so taxing on your muscles. Pay special attention to your hip flexors (the muscles in the crease at the front of your hip) and upper back muscles.

Time: Beginner: 5–15 minutes
Intermediate: 10–25 minutes
Advanced: 15–40 minutes

Areas targeted: Shoulders, Chest, Lower Back, Upper Back, Core, Upper Leg, Lower Leg

Props: Stability Ball

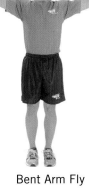

Shoulder Roll

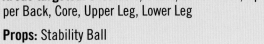

Bent Arm Fly

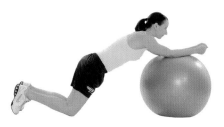

Stability Ball Reach

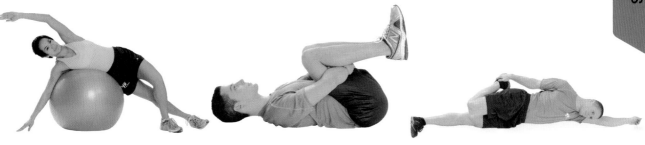

Lying Side Reach   Double Knees to Chest   Lying Side Quadriceps Stretch

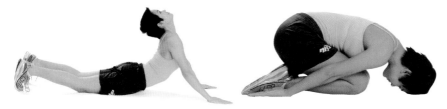

Lying Chest Lift (Cobra)   Child's Pose

Swimming

Although swimming gives you the benefit of a no-impact exercise, it's demanding in the fact that it encompasses practically every muscle in the body. Focus on the primary muscles involved with your stroke and be sure to include the muscles in the shoulders (front and back), chest, upper and lower back, and the triceps on the back of the upper arm.

Time: Beginner: 5–15 minutes
Intermediate: 10–25 minutes
Advanced: 15–40 minutes

Areas targeted: Neck, Shoulders, Arms, Chest, Upper Back, Hips, Lower Legs

Props: Stability Ball

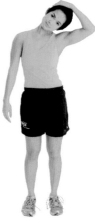

Side Neck Stretch

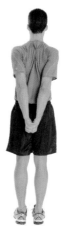

Behind Back Shoulder Reach

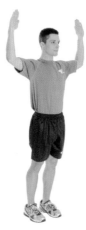

Standing Rotator Cuff

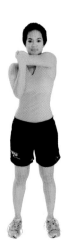

Bent Arm Triceps Crossover

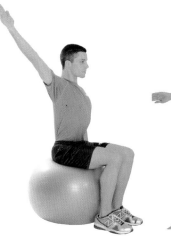

Seated Single Arm Chest Stretch

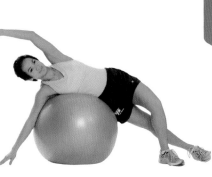

Lying Side Reach

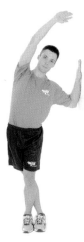

Standing Outer Hip Stretch

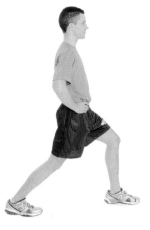

Standing Calf Stretch

Skiing

Skiing requires good balance, strength, and endurance. The more flexibility and elasticity you have in your muscles, the better they can perform and the quicker they can recover. Whether you're downhill or cross-country skiing, your back, glutes, and core muscles all play a major role in how well your legs can control the skis.

Time: Beginner: 5–15 minutes
Intermediate: 10–25 minutes
Advanced: 15–40 minutes

Areas targeted: Neck, Shoulders, Upper Back, Lower Back, Hips, Lower Legs

Props: Stability Ball

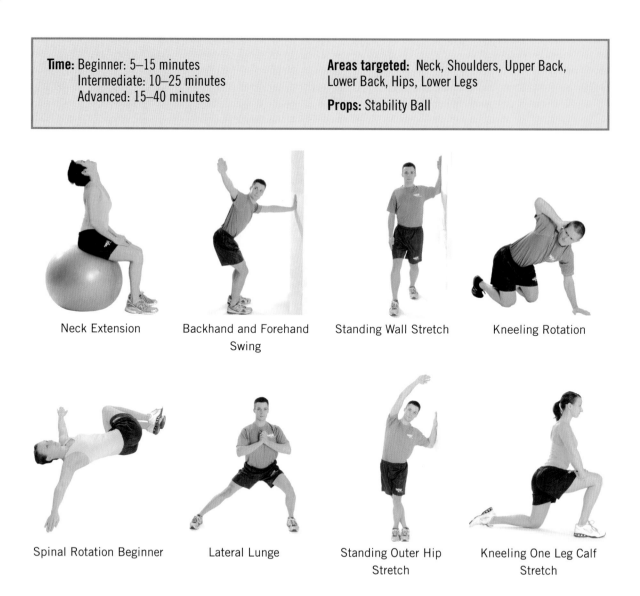

Neck Extension

Backhand and Forehand Swing

Standing Wall Stretch

Kneeling Rotation

Spinal Rotation Beginner

Lateral Lunge

Standing Outer Hip Stretch

Kneeling One Leg Calf Stretch

Cycling

Cycling is a repetitive exercise, and your hip, knee, and ankle never go through their full range of motion. It's a recipe for muscle fatigue, stiffness, and injury. To make matters worse, many cyclists spend countless hours a week in a crouched position, shortening the hip flexors. This can cause an anterior pelvic tilt and excessively arched lower back. Like runners, cyclists can benefit from yoga poses. Your overall flexibility routine should focus on reversing the cycling position.

Time: Beginner: 5–15 minutes
Intermediate: 10–25 minutes
Advanced: 15–40 minutes

Areas targeted: Shoulders, Upper Back, Lower Back, Core, Hips, Upper Leg

Props: Stability Ball, Risers

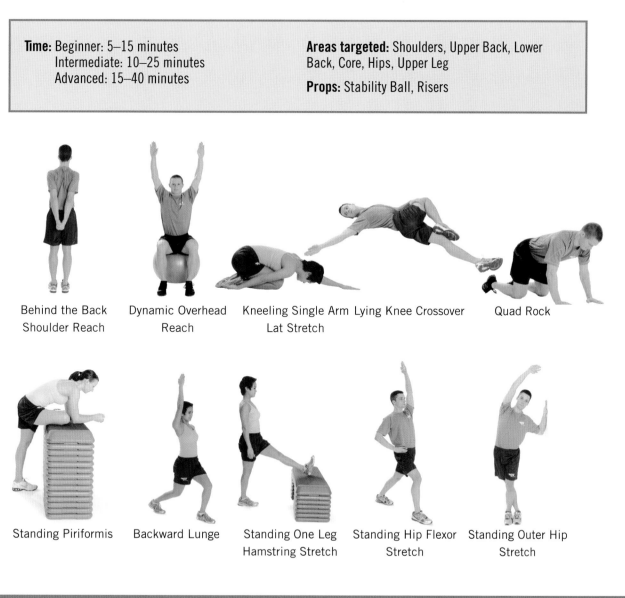

Behind the Back Shoulder Reach

Dynamic Overhead Reach

Kneeling Single Arm Lat Stretch

Lying Knee Crossover

Quad Rock

Standing Piriformis

Backward Lunge

Standing One Leg Hamstring Stretch

Standing Hip Flexor Stretch

Standing Outer Hip Stretch

Tennis

Have a game plan to prepare your body for a match before you step onto the court. After a light warm-up of hitting, it's good to begin with dynamic movements targeting your legs, trunk and arms. Lunges and rotations are key movements—and jumping jacks even hit the mark. After your match, while your muscles are still warm, is the ideal time to complete the static stretches in this section.

Time: Beginner: 5–15 minutes
Intermediate: 10–25 minutes
Advanced: 15–40 minutes

Areas targeted: Wrists, Shoulders, Upper Back, Hips, Lower Leg

Props: None

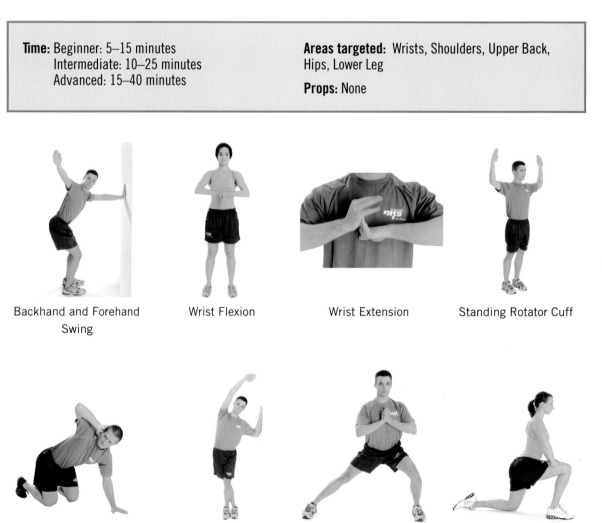

Backhand and Forehand Swing

Wrist Flexion

Wrist Extension

Standing Rotator Cuff

Kneeling Rotation

Standing Outer Hip Stretch

Lateral Lunge

Kneeling One Leg Calf Stretch

Golf

The first step to a full and fluid golf swing is good flexibility. Walking around the course before you start your dynamic movements is a good warm-up. The shoulders, low back, and hamstrings are the common problem areas for golfers, but don't neglect your forearms and wrists. After a round of golf, but before you leave the course, is an ideal time to complete the static stretches in this section.

Time: Beginner: 5–15 minutes
Intermediate: 10–25 minutes
Advanced: 15–40 minutes

Areas targeted: Wrists, Shoulders, Upper Back, Lower Back, Hips

Props: Dowel Rod, Ball

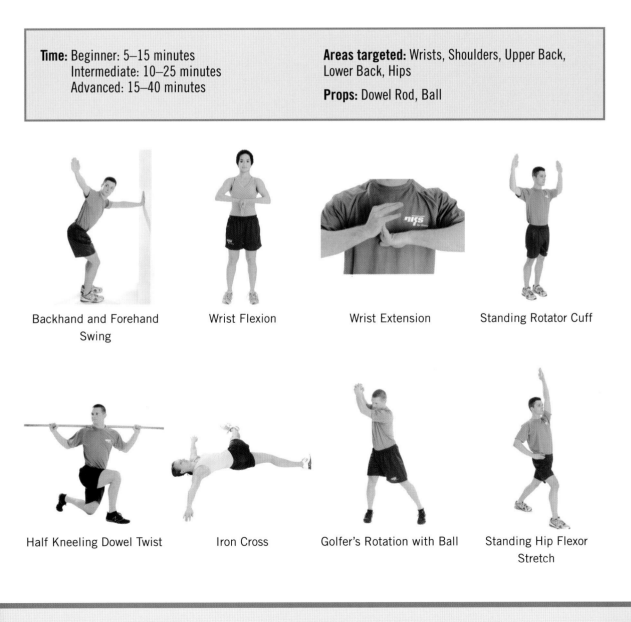

Backhand and Forehand Swing

Wrist Flexion

Wrist Extension

Standing Rotator Cuff

Half Kneeling Dowel Twist

Iron Cross

Golfer's Rotation with Ball

Standing Hip Flexor Stretch

Bowling

The long stride and sliding action of bowling place a toll on your lower body and back. It's important to be warm and loose and have ample range of motion before you start. Remember to stretch both sides of your body for muscle balance and coordination. Begin with dynamic movements for your hips, legs, and shoulders and then move on to specific stretches to target the lower body and shoulder.

Time: Beginner: 5–15 minutes
Intermediate: 10–25 minutes
Advanced: 15–40 minutes

Areas targeted: Wrists, Shoulders, Upper Back, Core, Hips

Props: None

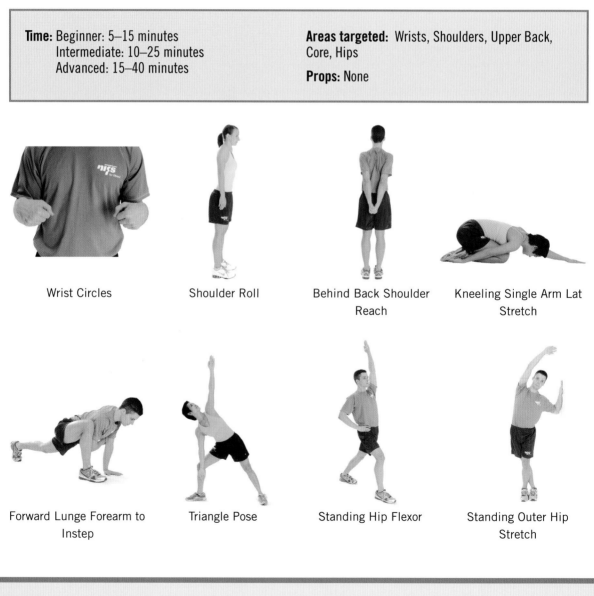

Wrist Circles

Shoulder Roll

Behind Back Shoulder Reach

Kneeling Single Arm Lat Stretch

Forward Lunge Forearm to Instep

Triangle Pose

Standing Hip Flexor

Standing Outer Hip Stretch

Basketball

Very few sports are as physically demanding as basketball. This sport is a continuous series of jumps, sprints, stops, twists, and turns. You must be able to move in every direction around the court. This requires abundant mobility in the hips and torso. Since your muscles must be flexible and responsive before they can be strong and explosive, the stretches in this routine focus on your torso, hips, quadriceps, and hamstrings.

Time: Beginner: 10–15 minutes
Intermediate: 15–25 minutes
Advanced: 20–40 minutes

Areas targeted: Shoulders, Chest, Core, Upper Back, Lower Back, Hips, Upper Legs, Lower Legs

Props: Foam Roller, Rope

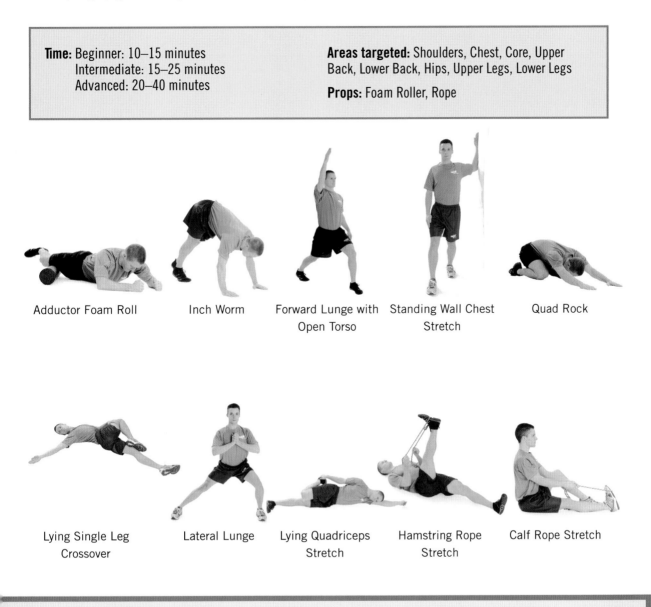

Adductor Foam Roll

Inch Worm

Forward Lunge with Open Torso

Standing Wall Chest Stretch

Quad Rock

Lying Single Leg Crossover

Lateral Lunge

Lying Quadriceps Stretch

Hamstring Rope Stretch

Calf Rope Stretch

Weight Lifting (Upper Body)

Weight lifting leaves your muscles feeling tight due to the constant contractions and the rush of blood to the area. The overload effect can also create micro tears in the muscle that leave you sore and stiff. A thorough warm-up, including dynamic stretches, and more targeted stretching during your weight lifting workout will help minimize the negatives and speed up your recovery. Pay extra attention to any area that doesn't seem in sync.

Time: Beginner: 5–15 minutes
Intermediate: 10–25 minutes
Advanced: 15–40 minutes

Areas targeted: Shoulders, Chest, Arms, Upper Back, Lower Back

Props: None

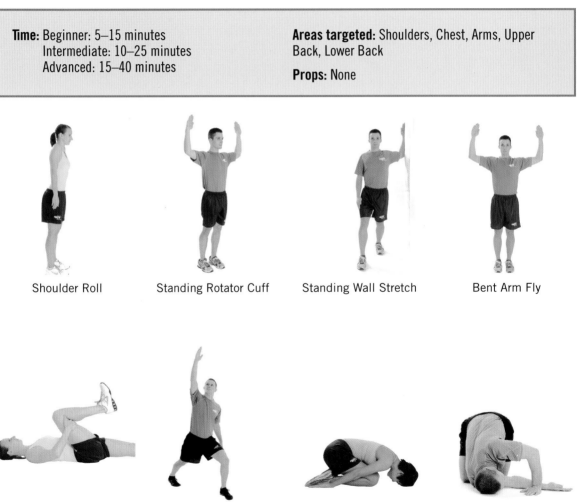

Shoulder Roll

Standing Rotator Cuff

Standing Wall Stretch

Bent Arm Fly

Single Knee to Chest

Forward Lunge with Open Trunk

Child's Pose

Kneeling Thread the Needle

Weight Lifting (Lower Body)

Lower body movements are usually compound movements that involve more than one joint and target multiple muscle groups. The muscles in the hips, quadriceps, and hamstrings are the body's biggest power generators, and the abdominals and low back muscles are often the stabilizers. After a 10-minute warm-up, perform dynamic movements to engage all the muscles from your trunk to your toes. During your workout, perform a few moderate reps of dynamic stretches between sets to keep your muscles loose.

Time: Beginner: 5–15 minutes
Intermediate: 10–25 minutes
Advanced: 15–40 minutes

Areas targeted: Lower Back, Upper Leg, Lower Leg, Hips

Props: Risers

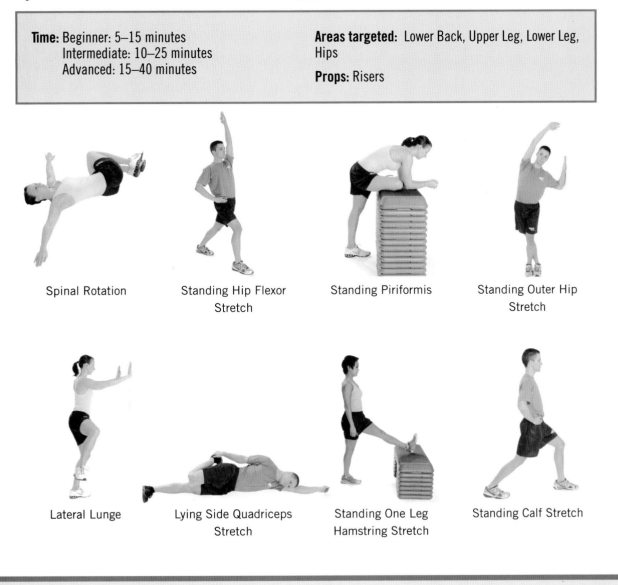

Spinal Rotation

Standing Hip Flexor Stretch

Standing Piriformis

Standing Outer Hip Stretch

Lateral Lunge

Lying Side Quadriceps Stretch

Standing One Leg Hamstring Stretch

Standing Calf Stretch

Advanced Stretching

The following stretches and poses integrate strength, stability, and balance. Not everyone is designed for every movement, so look for modifications to poses that don't feel right for you—or you might go only to the halfway point. If one stretch doesn't feel right, back off and try another. Be aware of areas that may be over flexible, as this leads to a weak and unstable joint. In the case of hyper-flexibility, strengthening, rather than stretching, may be needed.

Time: Beginner: 5–15 minutes
Intermediate: 10–25 minutes
Advanced: 15–40 minutes

Areas targeted: Upper Back, Lower Back, Core, Hips, Whole Body

Props: Stability Ball

Spinal Rotation Advanced

Advanced Piriformis Stretch

Stability Ball Back Release

Inch Worm

Reverse 90/90 Advanced

Bent Knee Side Angle Pose

Triangle Pose

Warrior 1

Warrior 2